CONTENTS

Introduction

Nothing's sadder than a runner who can't run. At any one time, there are a lot of sad runners. Some studies say that 50 percent of runners every year get injured enough so they can't run, while others say it's as much as 80 percent.

I was sad and desperate the day I walked into the Santa Monica, California, office of Forster Physical Therapy, the go-to fix-it shop for West L.A.'s runners, cyclists, and adventure racers. It was April 1999, 2 weeks before the Boston Marathon. I'd planned to run it, had purchased a plane ticket months before, but had a problem: I'd only done a total of 20 miles (32 km) in the previous 4 months because of intense, searing pain in my left hip when I ran. During that time, I'd already gone to several physical therapists, who typically had me do a series of pelvic stretching exercises; these did not solve the problem at all.

But Robert Forster, a PT-to-the-stars known for treating some of the biggest names in running, tennis, and other sports, starting with Florence "Flo-Jo" Griffith Joyner and Jackie Joyner-Kersee at the 1984 and 1988 Olympics, approached my hip pain differently. He didn't mention stretching at all (that would come later). He had me jog up and down the hallway for 10 seconds. Then he said this:

"You have excessive side-to-side body sway that is torquing your hip; that's probably what's causing the pain. To stop the sway, try swinging your arms vertically alongside your rib cage, not sideways across your chest." Until that moment, I had no idea that my arms did not swing vertically.

Forster wasn't done yet. "As for your crazy fantasy of finishing a marathon on no training, you have no hope whatsoever of doing that unless . . . "

"Unless what?" I said.

"Unless you completely change your form—*right now*. Listen and repeat after me: 'High knees, proper arm swing, and rapid turnover. This will shorten your stride and force your feet to land under the center of your body. Run softly. No heel strike.' Your goal: Baby your body and reduce the impact on your joints by distributing the load over more, smaller steps. Forget long strides: You fly through the air farther, crash down hard on your heel, and put more leverage and stress on your muscles and tendons, leading to injuries. If you don't baby your untrained muscles with short strides in Boston, you'll flame out long before you reach the finish line."

Then Forster gave me a visual: "You want to be like the Road Runner, legs underneath you, circling in a blur, feet barely touching the ground. Beep-beep!"

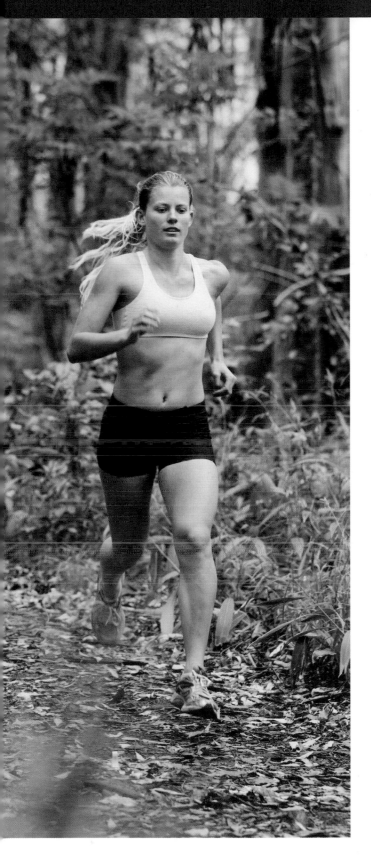

Completely change my form? Short strides? Vertical arm swing? Baby my body? I'd never heard any of this before. Hardly anyone had— it was a decade before *Born to Run* put the spotlight on running injuries and the relationship between them and poor running mechanics. But unbeknownst to me, what Forster described was the way the best runners in the world ran, and that's who he had learned it from, literally starting the day that he graduated physical therapy school.

Studying with a cutting-edge team of running-biomechanics experts at Centinela Hospital Medical Center in Los Angeles, Forster quickly became the running expert at the world-renowned Kerlan-Jobe Clinic, which took care of sports teams, such as the Lakers, Kings, and Rams. Forster then traveled to international running events around the globe with a young, soon-to-be-famous UCLA coach named Bob Kersee as they trained a team that would go on to win forty-six medals at the next eight Olympic Games. When Forster opened his own practice in 1983 (as well as his Phase IV Scientific Health & Performance Center in 2003), he applied the same rules to regular folks that he learned from the elites: Good form and gradual adaptation make for a fitter, stronger, faster, and less-injured athlete.

When I left Forster's office that April morning in 1999, armed with my Road Runner imagery, I headed right to a treadmill at my gym. In minutes, I received the most pleasant shock of my life: no pain in my hip while running for the first time in years!

Suddenly, my Boston experiment didn't seem so impossible. The hardest part was done! Over the next 10 days, I logged 34 training miles (54.4 km), maxed out with a 13-miler (20.8 km), cross-trained on the elliptical, and flew east. From my first steps at the 103rd Boston Marathon, I religiously stuck to my little Road Runner strides. I was too afraid not to. As Forster had advised, I didn't push it. I focused on my pendulum arm swing and little pin-wheeling stride. Through 10, 15, 20 miles (16, 24, 32 km), it worked perfectly. I climbed Heartbreak Hill without a twinge. Then, overexcited by my success with my new form, I forgot about it. Forster's advice was out the window as I lengthened my strides and flung my feet way ahead of my body on the long gradual downhill into mile 24. That's where the chaos began, as it had to. The last 2 spasm-wracked miles weren't pretty, but I stumbled across the finish in 3:56—to the amazement of my friends, who'd all bet I'd be on the bus by mile 16.

I was amazed, too. Just finishing that day changed forever how I thought about running. If shorter strides and a vertical arm swing was this easy on your body in a marathon, imagine how much healthier and less injured you'd be if you ran this way over a lifetime. And you'd probably run faster, too. If I'd had more time to train, I would have shattered my personal record.

When I came home and told Forster that, and thanked him endlessly for what he'd done for me, he slapped me on the back.

"Exactly! Performance, injury prevention, and injury rehab are all linked," he said. "You can't separate them! That's what I've been preaching for years!"

Forster believes that you can't just fix an injury in isolation. When I came in with my hip injury, it wasn't my hip that was causing the problem, it was a bigger-picture issue. "A good PT isn't just an auto mechanic who fixes a worn part," he says. "You have to figure out what's causing the wear. So he also has to be an investigator who hunts around and finds the root of the problem upstream. Fix the cause, and you get fewer injuries and less downtime—meaning better training and better results."

This is why Forster takes a holistic view of addressing running injuries, and why we divided *Healthy Running Step By Step* into two parts:

Section 1:

A big-picture game plan that can stop injuries from happening in the first place, starting with a time-tested "Periodization" training plan to gradually adapt your body to race distances while remaining injury-free, and a full-body assessment of your flexibility, strength, posture, balance, and training history.

Section 2:

A pain-relief rehab program that will nurse you back to full strength with a graduated series of adaptations. Over the years, Forster has designed a template of actions for every major running injury that you will see here as a large grid, labeled Self-Diagnosis and Rehab Matrix.

Most PTs ignore section 1 and skip right to section 2. Forster addresses section 1 first to improve running mechanics, train to prevent injuries, keep runners out of rehab, and stop the problem from happening again.

Assessment, Prevention, and Rehab

In an ideal world, you wouldn't wait until you get injured to fix your problems. That inevitably leads to re-injury and a return trip to rehab. To prevent the physical therapy yo-yo, you'd "fix" your injuries *before* they even happen, starting with learning proper form (such as eliminating arm cross-chest swings and heel striking). Another key chapter discusses balance and posture, which get corrupted over the years by a host of stresses that wreck side-to-side symmetry. Everyone, whether they know it or not, has certain mechanical issues, such as leg-length discrepancies (a widespread problem that affects most people); previous traumatic injury weaknesses and dominant-/weak-side body imbalances; joint and collagen degeneration from

age or disease; and medicine-induced deterioration to joints and collagen.

This is where weight training and stretching come in. Covered in substantial chapters, they are each necessary to build and maintain speed, ensure healthy running again, and help keep the body aligned and symmetrical.

That's especially important for runners, because running as we practice it in the modern world magnifies the smallest misalignments and imbalances. "If you can imagine that humans are 'primal' beings who evolved into our current form over a few million years, you have to recognize that exercise as we know it today isn't what hunter-gatherers did," says Forster. "They didn't go 22 or 23 hours without moving, then bolt off on a heart-throbbing run for 45 minutes, like we do today. They did a variety of stuff—long, fast marches to chase big game, short sprints to dodge tusks or spears, and slow walking to gather berries. Their bodies were strong and their tendons and ligaments hardened by constant movement, so misaligned joints could handle the stress. But when subjected to daily bouts of intense, repetitive motion, like modern running, stress and wear are accelerated—and runners have to come see people like me."

In other words, modern running is an inherently risky activity. Add a work ethic that encourages you to push hard all the time without proper rest and recovery, and the sport almost

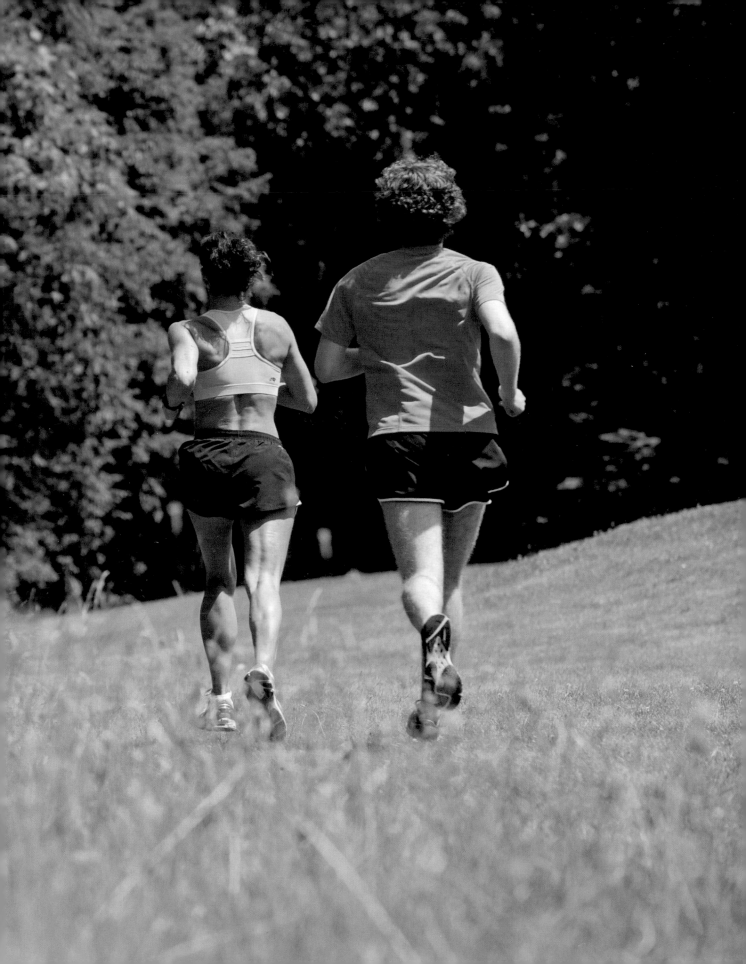

wills you into overtraining, a condition in which muscles and joints receive no time to heal after hard workouts. At best, most runners I meet are always somewhat fatigued, making them vulnerable to illness and injury. It's no surprise that most of them get sick or hurt.

That's why following a classic Periodization training schedule is so important. Periodization, in case you haven't heard of it, is a training schedule used by the world's best strength and aerobic athletes for decades to gradually and safely ramp up your fitness. It incrementally increases your running volume to build your base, backs off every few weeks temporarily to allow recovery, and then adds more strength and speed work to sharpen you up for your 10k or marathon.

If you get Periodization right, it eliminates overtraining and the injuries that result from it. But if your running program is designed by your daily whim and allowed to get stale without intelligent progression, you will end up burned out, injured, or both.

Other chapters in section 1 also tell you how to identify signs of overtraining, so you can avoid it, and provide a tutorial on postexercise recovery techniques such as icing, compression, and elevation, so that you can come back next time even stronger and faster.

The instructions in section 2, *Healthy Running Step By Step*'s rehab program, focus on the "big 5" running injuries: IT band syndrome,

Achilles tendonitis, shin splints, plantar fasciitis, and hamstring strains.

For each of the five injuries, Forster developed a Self-Diagnosis and Rehab Matrix that asks you to assess your own injury and its severity, with an 8-week time frame for the worst ones. It then takes you through your rehab step-by-step, from the bread-and-butter physical therapy protocol of PRICE (protection, rest, ice, compression, elevation) to simple range-of-motion movements, strengthening and stretching exercises, cross-training activities, and finally, regular running and hill work.

The matrix is so comprehensive and logical that in many cases you will be able to rehab yourself. If you choose to visit a PT, the chapter information and matrix will educate you well enough to have a say in your treatment.

SUMMARY: THINK LONG-TERM

We know that most readers of this book will immediately turn to the injury rehab matrix to get pain relief and a quick recuperation to get back to their regular running routine. But they shouldn't forget what caused the injury in the first place.

"Early in my career, I would start at the injury rehab matrix when dealing with patients," says Forster. "But then I realized that fixing mechanics and creating a sound training program, with attention to proper mechanics, stretching, strengthening, and diet, are more important, almost preventing the need for the matrix." With this philosophy in mind, we laid out the book by placing preventive, long-term measures up front.

Injuries are a risk in all sports and seemingly a part of the job description for runners, who have chosen a strenuous, repetitive activity that has a tendency to exaggerate leg-length discrepancies, old injury sites, and all biomechanical inefficiencies to the point where they create injuries. Forster, educated by decades of treating thousands of patients, from Olympians to 80-year-olds, has learned that the most important aspect of treatment is a big-picture view that uncovers (and fixes) the causes of the injuries so they won't come back. That's why we spend a lot of time describing a joint-friendly running form and an organized, gradual, and safe Periodized training plan, augmented by regular stretching and strength work that helps your body retain symmetry and buttress weak spots. With this approach, most running injuries are avoidable. If you're not injured yet, make section 1 your bible.

If you do get injured, it is important to participate in rehabilitation with a long-term solution to the problem in mind. Otherwise, you'll soon be riding the rehab yo-yo back to your PT. Study the specific injury's exclusive Self-Diagnosis and Rehab Matrix. Each one lays out a schedule for full recovery. Don't rush it. Spend your downtime wisely by reading about the importance of improving posture, strength, and flexibility, all described in the following pages. Then get a head start on those tasks while you rehabilitate your whole body, keeping in mind the big picture of health and performance.

SECTION 1: A Long-Term Guide to Injury Prevention and Peak Performance

1 Why Runners Get Hurt

Injuries are inevitable due to overuse, lack of recovery, poor diet, lousy form, and failure to shore up your infrastructure and create a fat-burning engine. Here, Bob Forster explains how to keep your running safe.

One of the most basic rules of sports medicine is, "You need 2 days off from running for every day that you've run in pain." So if you've felt some pain for a week, then you should not run for 2 weeks. If all you remember from this book is that rule, you might add decades to your running career.

It became clear to me in my first years as a physical therapist that most running injuries are actually overuse injuries, and they take a long time to develop. It's much easier to understand and treat an acute injury. But repetitive motion injuries that create inflammation (discussed in "The Anatomy of Overtraining Injuries" on pages 22–23) and accumulate scar tissue over months and years can't be addressed with a quick fix. It doesn't matter whether you're an elite runner or a back-of-the-packer—you have probably ignored an injury for way too long, to your detriment.

In 1978, when I first began treating runners, they were seen as an enigmatic group of loners who spent hours of solitude slogging through longer and longer workouts. Finding solitude became harder as millions more laced up running shoes over the years, motivated by the health benefits of regular exercise and the simplicity and economy of the sport. After all, running was easy and required little investment in goods or

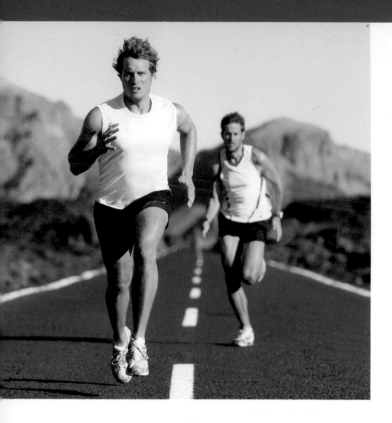

coaching. Everyone already "knew" how to run: just like they did as kids.

After a few years, the exhilaration that comes with the repetitive cyclic motion of running was identified as the *runner's high*. The exhilaration was also tied to the release of morphine-like chemicals in the brain called *endorphins*. Runners didn't really understand endorphins, but they knew they made them feel good. Before long, millions of runners were hooked. They ran every day, through rain and cold and even snow.

Back then no one knew how to stretch—or how to buy shoes. There were only a few brands on the market with limited choices. They didn't know pronation from supination or why it mattered. Their social group outside running shrank

down in size because their friends thought they were a bit crazy, and their spouses and family felt left out—but none of this stopped runners from running. They defended their fanatical dedication to running by citing literature that promised near immortality from the cardiovascular health benefits of aerobic exercise. Hard-core runners, so caught up in their addictive overtraining, seemed to believe that one missed day of running would clog their arteries overnight and they would die of heart disease.

It was therefore inevitable that the only thing that would stop obsessed runners who did not yet know that too much of a good thing is bad would be injury. By the mid-'80s, too many runners landed in my physical therapy office in Santa Monica with severe and debilitating injuries. Why? Because they ran too much, too often, and too far. They came in the office with bags of running shoes whose wear pattern they hoped would provide an answer to their chronic injury pattern. In an attempt to manage the fanatical allegiance to their sport, many doctors were reluctant to tell runners to stop running. It was the ignorant leading the obsessed; soon, shin splints turned into stress fractures, heel bones grew bone spurs, and running through injuries caused irreversibly damaged tendons.

I know this firsthand because I became one of them. As a former college wrestler from New York who needed to find a transition sport to

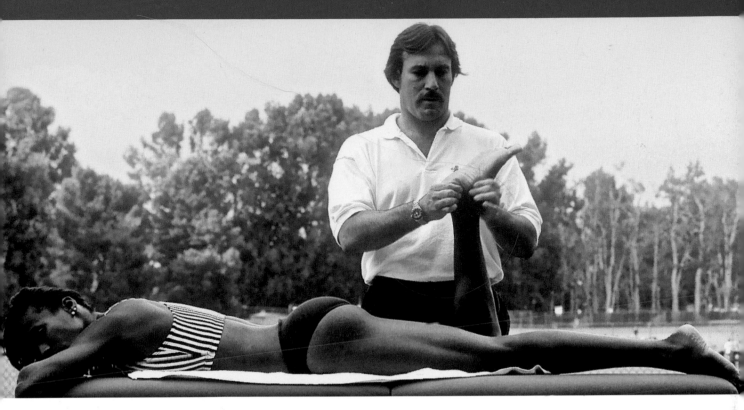

Robert Forster, P.T., working on three-time Olympic gold medalist Jackie Joyner-Kersee before the 1992 Olympics.

feed my need to stay fit, the sun-drenched bike path along Santa Monica beach was too alluring to avoid falling prey to the running obsession.

Only months after beginning to run, I built my mileage up to marathon-training volume and I unwisely ran two marathons in the first year. I was hooked now, too. Even as a freshly minted physical therapist who knew better, I couldn't keep myself from running through pain. Suffering chronic shin splints, I applied physical therapy treatment to my aching legs and did exercises to strengthen the sore tendons to the point where I could move a small house with my ankle inverters. I even got fitted for orthotic devices in my shoes. But still the pain persisted, because my vision was too limited.

Although we clinicians were proficient at identifying common running injuries, the focus of clinical treatment remained reactive and not proactive. The treatment for foot or leg injuries was orthotic devices or an exercise or two in an attempt to strengthen the overburdened tendons. The problem was that the source of the injury, which can be remote from the painful area, was not addressed.

At the same time I was working with one of the most successful running coaches in the world, Bob Kersee, and I began to think there was a better approach. My work with Kersee and his elite track and field athletes changed my treatment focus to address the mechanics of the whole athlete. When I changed my approach and instructed runners in proper running technique, and then used stretching and strengthening exercises that facilitated those good mechanics, the new approach served to normalize and reduce the forces that bore down on the commonly injured tissues of the lower extremities and pelvis. With correct running mechanics, along with a bit of local treatment for the injured structures, runners not only got past their current painful condition, but started to break the chronic injury-reinjury cycle.

In the ensuing decade, a body of scientific research began to reveal the physiological adaptations needed to transition from couch potato to runner. Slowly, training programs based on science and not obsession were emerging as we learned how to train for the specific adaptations needed for injury-free, peak performance. We learned the necessity of rest days, the value of stretching to reverse the natural shortening of connective tissues that is accelerated with running, the importance of increasing mileage slowly, and the role of differently constructed running shoes to match foot types.

Runners changed, too. By the mid-'90s, more runners were cross-training and spreading the stress of their workouts over more joints of the body. Soon many runners became triathletes and adventure racers; the more balanced training helped them become fitter and avoid injury. The loneliness of the long distance runner began to erode as running clubs emerged with a less

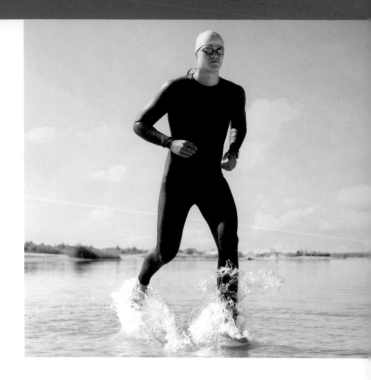

fanatical devotion to back-to-back hard workouts and weeks and months of high mileage.

So why then do runners still get injured so often? After years of treating runners, I have found that the same personality traits that attract individuals to choose running often work against them and lead them to injury.

PROBLEM #1: Runners Don't See the Big Picture

Some runners hate the gym but love to stretch. Some hate both stretching and weight training. And most seem to think that because they work out so much, they can eat whatever they like.

Too often I meet runners who fall in love with running but pick and choose from the other aspects of training that they need to keep them running injury-free. This is especially true for those not focused on performance, who don't necessarily care whether they get on the podium because they just run for the love of it.

Well, the fact is that runners can't just run—and they can't cherry-pick. To keep your running injury-free, stay healthy, and protect against common running injuries that can sideline you for a while or end your running career, and alter your lifestyle, you have to do *all* the things that you may not like doing, such as stretching, lifting weights, eating better, and correcting your running mechanics. These four training variables—structural integrity, metabolic efficiency, nutritional optimization, and running technique—are no secret, because the healthiest, most successful athletes do them. I've come to call them the Four Pillars of Health and Performance.

Over the years, as I scrutinized the most successful athletic programs anywhere—for example, USC football, the Los Angeles Lakers, and, most of all, Bob Kersee's track and field group—it has become clear that they were successful year after year because they stayed focused on all of the Four Pillars. Ignore any of them for too long, and you will run into problems.

For instance, if you don't improve your structural integrity—the strength and flexibility of joints, bones, muscles, and connective tissue—you will be unable to perform correct running mechanics, and eventually overburden your body as it struggles to withstand excessive forces. If you don't pay attention to your metabolic efficiency—particularly the ability to use fat as a major fuel source for running—you will fatigue early in your workout and risk injury, as your deteriorating muscle function causes you to suffer strains and sprains. Ditto if you don't optimize your nutrition to support your training and recovery efforts. And the best-trained and -fed runner can still wreck his joints without adopting the proper running technique.

Bottom line: You can't run in isolation or train just some of the Four Pillars and expect not to break down. You have to pay some attention to each of these key areas of training. Ideally, you work them simultaneously.

SOLUTION: Work All Four Pillars of Health and Performance throughout the Training Cycle

The Four Pillars not only provide the framework for performance, injury prevention, and weight management, but the reduction of health risk factors. These are the same aspects of health that all citizens, not just athletes, need to focus on to live long, healthy lives. Whether you are training for your first or fiftieth marathon, to get on the podium, or just to maintain your weight and preserve health, keeping all four key aspects of training in mind every week will keep you moving steadily toward your goal (see "The Four Pillars in the House of Health and Performance" on pages 16–17 for more details).

THE FOUR PILLARS IN THE HOUSE OF HEALTH AND PERFORMANCE

The foundation of the Four Pillars in the House of Health and Performance is recovery. Without it, all work is futile because it is during periods of rest that your fitness actually evolves. Governing all your training efforts is the psychology of healthy living and self-improvement.

1. STRUCTURAL INTEGRITY (STRENGTH AND FLEXIBILITY)

Structural integrity refers to how well the muscular and skeletal systems function to propel you forward and protect you against injury. This is a function of strength, flexibility, joint alignment, and the resiliency of tissues to withstand the repetitive stress of running. Structural integrity is best achieved with a progressive, science-based running program along with strength and flexibility training. The components of structural integrity are explained in chapters 4 and 5. Strength and flexibility are developed simultaneously with Pillar #2, metabolic efficiency, during Periodization training.

2. METABOLIC EFFICIENCY

The word *metabolism* describes the internal processes that turn food into usable energy needed for all bodily functions. The body uses carbohydrates and fats for energy (some protein as well, but only in small percentages). You establish metabolic efficiency by training at specific intensities to create a metabolism in which fat becomes the preferred fuel for exercise and daily activities. Fat is the best fuel for runners because it provides an almost unlimited supply of energy; the average person has more than 80,000 calories of stored fat. It burns clean without producing lactic acid, a harmful waste product of carbohydrates, and provides more energy per gram than carbs. Also, a fat-burning metabolism allows for less reliance on external energy sources during prolonged exercise, such as gels, bars, and energy drinks. Limiting your reliance on these energy sources will help you avoid the most common source of failure in the marathon: gastrointestinal distress, including abdominal cramping, bloating, gas, and worse. Metabolic efficiency is explained in detail in chapter 5.

3. NUTRITIONAL OPTIMIZATION

Food should be thought of as fuel—the fuel needed to run your body. Nutritional optimization refers to how well you fuel your body for daily activities, workouts, and racing. By optimizing what and when you eat, nutrition will maintain your energy levels, increase your metabolic fitness, and help achieve your ideal body weight and performance goals. Effective sports nutrition starts with good daily nutrition, including consuming sufficient amounts of macro- and micronutrients every day.

A sound nutrition plan takes into account your activity level and food preferences. A sustainable eating plan is one that includes a variety of foods and can be maintained over time while providing adequate nutrients and achieving your optimal competition weight.

4. RUNNING TECHNIQUE

For every sport or fitness activity, proper technique ensures optimum maximum benefit, decreased injury, and improved performance.

Running technique is based on a few simple laws of physics. Your body must move in certain patterns to exploit the energy-saving aspects of these physical laws. Although our bodies were built for efficient running, our mostly sedentary lifestyles have robbed us of the ability to attain the most efficient mechanics. Technique training is the fastest, easiest, and most injury-free way to improve your times. Read about it in detail next in chapter 2.

FOUR PILLARS OF PERFORMANCE

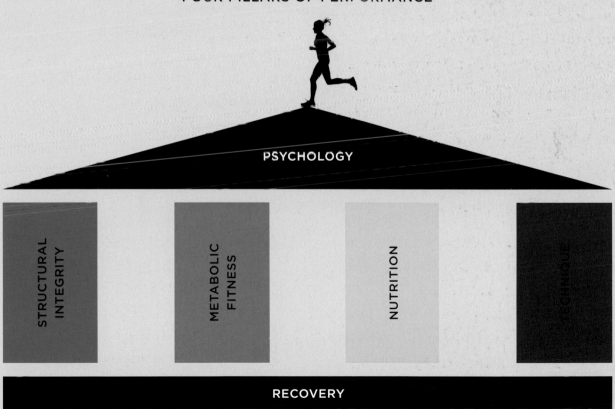

PSYCHOLOGY

STRUCTURAL INTEGRITY

METABOLIC FITNESS

NUTRITION

TECHNIQUE

RECOVERY

PROBLEM #2: Runners Are Too Competitive

The competitive streak in runners often drives them to increase mileage too quickly, push the pace too soon, and in general work too hard to achieve their goals. Runners are typically a highly motivated group, whether our goal is to achieve a respectable finish in the local 10k or a qualifying time for the Boston Marathon, or a more intrinsic goal to reach a specific weekly mileage, or finish a particularly long training run. This drive for achievement often clouds good judgment, and leads us to make decisions that are not productive. We push ourselves to run faster and farther than our body can tolerate and we become either overtrained, burned out, or both.

SOLUTION: Slow Down and Don't Ignore the Pain

If you feel pain in the same area during or after two runs in a 7- to 10-day period, consider yourself injured. Immediately cut your daily mileage in half, eliminate speed work and hills for 2 weeks, stretch more, and ice the injured area three times per day for 20 minutes with ice cubes and water, not a gel pack. After 2 weeks of recovery, slowly build up your mileage by no more than 10 percent per week and only add speed work and hills after you are back to your previous mileage pain-free. If pain persists, seek evaluation by a qualified physical therapist.

PROBLEM #3: You're a Dogmatic Do-It-Yourselfer

Runners don't want to rely on others to get their workouts in. Instead, running becomes a lifestyle in which workouts, along with all the preparation, nutrition, and recovery, need to be self-managed. Runners also want their performance to stand on its own, as running is typically not a team sport. This strong tendency for self-reliance will often lead runners to *try* to solve their own problems. Whether it is cramping or injury, runners will look within to heal their injuries, as opposed to relying on others. This self-reliance makes them reluctant to seek professional help until injuries become chronic.

SOLUTION: Ask for Help

A good coach, or at least a scientific training plan, will protect you from undermining your efforts with an overly rigid mind-set. Science-based training allows for recovery with built-in rest days and follows the hard-easy principle of training to allow your body the time it requires to adapt to the stress of your workouts. Science-based recovery strategies allow runners to direct their focus into restorative practices that will serve to make them more competitive on the roads and the track.

PROBLEM #4: You've Got Bad Form—and You Don't Know It

Runners view running as the most natural activity one can do for exercise. We all ran as kids whether or not we were athletes, so adults who take up running rarely seek instruction as they would if they took up golf or tennis. In a similar vein, runners can be reluctant to seek restorative therapies; they think injuries should heal naturally.

Well, the fact is that running injuries don't heal with rest alone. Because running is such a mechanical endeavor, injuries need to be addressed on a mechanical level. Unless the harsh G-forces (the accelerating forces of *gravity* that effectively multiply your body weight by three or four times at the point of a heel strike) that lead to injuries are redistributed, and the injured structure is unloaded, it doesn't matter if you take 3 weeks or 3 months off running. The tissue will break down again once you return to running if you have deficiencies in your running mechanics.

SOLUTION: Correct Your Mechanics

All overuse running injuries require you to make a change in the way your body is currently working. The key is to address the mechanical source of the injury with stretching and strengthening exercises to improve the way the joints function all along the kinetic chain. A slow return to running with corrected running mechanics has proven to be the best path for the injured runner.

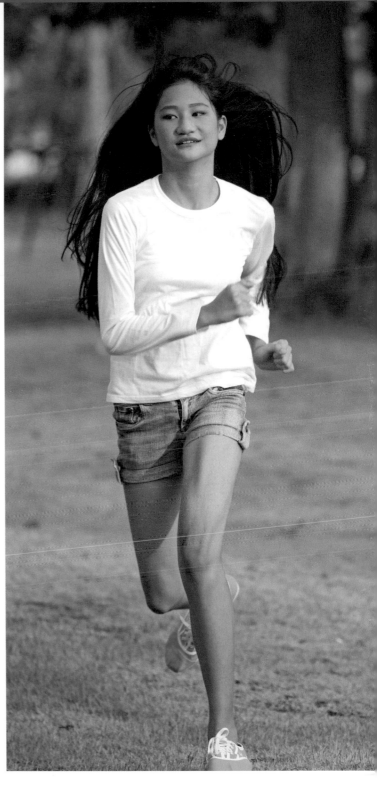

Note the cross-chest arm swing and faulty knock-kneed, or valgus alignment, of the lower extremity in this example of bad running form.

PROBLEM #5: Your Work Ethic Has Run Amok

Runners are not afraid of hard work. In fact, many think they need to suffer to get fit and actually expect that their body will hurt along the path to high performance. Unfortunately, this puts runners on a collision course with injury. The inability to discern good pain from bad pain becomes distorted, and soon one area of pain persists until the damaged structure can no longer withstand the workouts. That's when a runner's world begins to crumble. Taking time away from running to rest an injury can mean the loss of social group support and the psychological stress release that often helps them cope and function well in other areas of their life. Often the need to get back to running clouds good judgment—and their return is further delayed by reinjury.

SOLUTION: Relax, Recover, and Cross-Train

Drop the "no-pain, no-gain" mentality. Embrace recovery; always follow a hard day with an easy day and have a cross-training option available to replace running when injury strikes, allowing you to switch workouts to maintain your fitness and your sanity. While you work on improving the way your joints function with an active rehabilitation program and allow the injured structure to heal, you'll preserve your fitness, and in some cases, actually improve it.

PROBLEM #6: You've Turned Running into an Addiction

Do you run when you know it's going to make your injury or illness worse? Do you run even though your PT told you to bike and swim for your rehab? Do you try to sneak in a run when you know it'll make you late to pick up a relative at the airport or miss a work deadline? Do you run because you think running helps keep you focused on your other activities? Do you run because you've come to rely on the natural chemicals it produces to put you in a good mood, to cope with life?

If you answered "yes" to any of those, you are addicted to running. That's not all bad, unless you find that the running is controlling you instead of you controlling your running. If your exercise becomes self-destructive, you are out of balance.

SOLUTION: Find Other Therapy and Stick to a Training Plan

First, admit something's out of balance in your life. Don't make running your way of coping with your problems. Do you need meditation? Do you need medication? Or psychotherapy, yoga, or another hobby? Next, separate your running from your therapy by getting someone to write a Periodization training program for you. That way, your program will tell you when you should run, when you should rest, when to go hard, how to eat right, and when to lift weights.

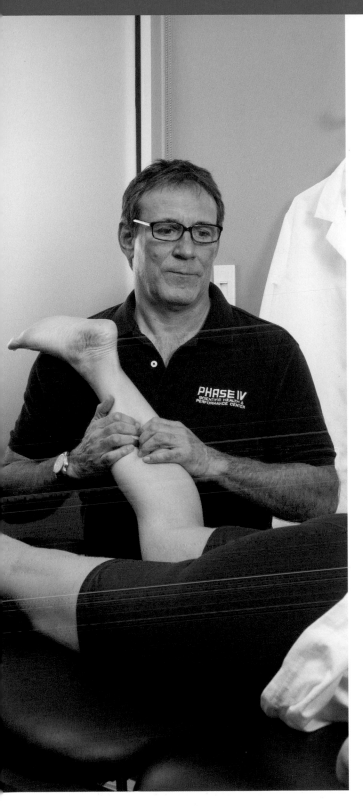

Find a sports physical therapist who has experience working with runners to treat your injury.

PROBLEM #7: You're Not Getting Good Medical Help

At the risk of sounding a bit self-serving, the fact is that it's hard to find doctors and therapists who are qualified to treat running injuries. All overuse running injuries are 100 percent mechanical in origin and therefore require clinicians who understand biomechanics and address them with a holistic approach. This means stretches over supplements, active exercises over little black boxes with dubious healing powers, and education over dogma. Those who take the time to understand the mechanics of good running form and how to facilitate it create effective treatment plans that make them active participants in their rehabilitation and not passive recipients of care.

SOLUTION: Find an Experienced Sports Physical Therapist

Find a physical therapist who works with runners by asking around and interviewing them on the phone regarding their approach to your ailment. Expect them to take a careful history and thorough physical examination of your alignment, flexibility, and strength and also evaluate your running mechanics before allowing you to return to running.

THE ANATOMY OF OVERTRAINING INJURIES:

CHRONIC INFLAMMATION, INCOMPLETE HEALING, AND LACK OF RECOVERY

Unless you fall down and break a bone or step wrong and sprain your ankle, the vast majority of running injuries you are likely to suffer are overuse injuries. Overuse injuries occur when we outpace our body's ability to adapt to the stress of training. The micro-trauma suffered by the tissues during training, which would normally heal and make us stronger with adequate recovery (the foundation of the Four Pillars in the House of Health and Performance), instead builds into a macro-trauma with back-to-back hard days and weeks of training.

By the time pain arises, the typical overuse injury may be weeks or months in the making. The injured tissue most likely had been struggling to heal for quite some time, but the repetitive stress of running stalled the healing process.

The chain of physiological events that is put in motion to repair the damaged tissues begins with the inflammatory response. This is a characteristic reaction set in motion to first clean up the debris of the damaged cells and then begin the healing of the injured area with scar tissue.

These events are repeated throughout your body every time you run, and they go unnoticed if your training is progressive and designed with built-in time for recovery—and that means several recovery days every week, a recovery week every month, and some time off every year. You see, when your workouts are too frequent, or too hard, and go on for too long and without meaningful variation or enough time provided for recovery, the body struggles to stay ahead of the stress.

If the healing process from the microtrauma is incomplete and the scar tissue has not matured enough to withstand the stress of your next workout, it gets broken down and the process starts all over again. The problem then becomes one of excess scar tissue and chronic inflammation. The inflammation leads to scar tissue, and the scar tissue causes dysfunction in the injured structure, which propagates more tissue damage and chronic inflammation, the inflammation causes pain, and the pain causes muscle tightness or spasm and more dysfunction in a circular downward spiral that eventually stops you in your tracks.

Face it: Running is so addictive that even the most self-aware disciple of Periodization training can slip into overtraining and pick up an overuse injury if he or she gets a little distracted. That's why it's so important to be aware of the signs of overtraining, which include sleepless nights, weight gain or loss, frequent illness, and chronic injury—and then to do something about it. Step one in the recovery process is simple logic: Halt the damaging workouts. Then, find a pain-free cross-training modality and address the inflammation with aggressive icing. Next, relieve the muscle tightness with stretching and break up scar tissue with the foam roller or cross-fiber friction massage by a qualified professional.

The key is when you feel an injury developing, don't delay. The sooner you start the recovery process, and address the mechanical cause, the sooner you'll be back on the road.

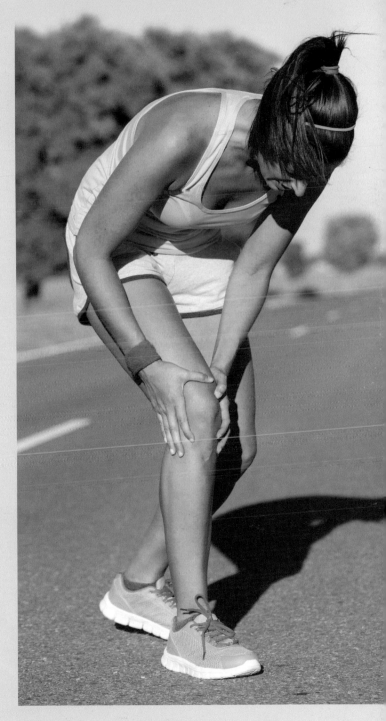

Chronic inflammation can lead to muscle tightness or spasm.

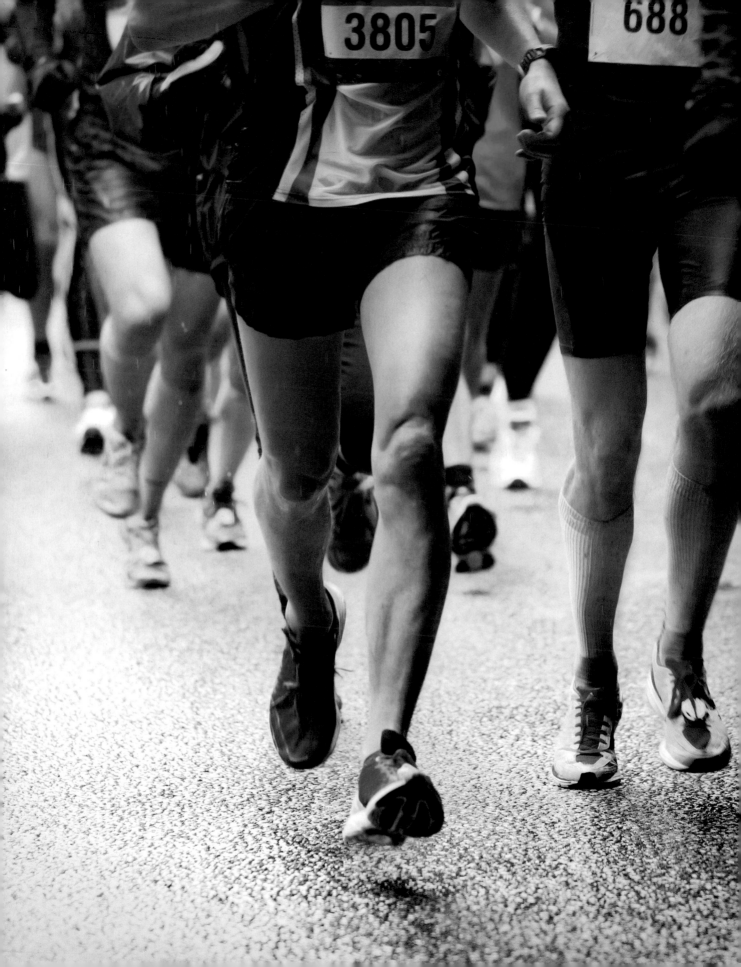

2 Technique and Shoes

Three simple form changes will add speed and end the debilitating heel strike.

We humans are movement machines. Evolution built our bodies to run, walk, and stride for long distances at fast speeds, probably to track down animals for dinner—and run from them when they have other ideas. Compared to our slower primate cousins, human bodies have a large number of running-friendly features: shorter arms to balance the cyclic movement of the legs; lighter lower legs and thicker hips, which allow the leg to swing with little effort like a pendulum; bigger, more complex feet, to absorb shock; and thicker lumbar vertebrae, also to absorb greater shock forces. In addition, we have a built-in economy of motion that turns our muscles, tendons, and connective tissue into natural springs, slings, and pendulums that effectively store energy during the gait cycle, then return it on the next step.

So if we are natural runners, why do we so often get hurt doing it?

The trouble is that the sedentary lifestyle of the modern world has basically ruined our ability to exploit our gifts. Unburdened of the need to hunt and chase and carry, we don't move enough and have become soft. As with everything related to the body, it's a case of "use it or lose it." Even though you run 1 hour a day, in the modern world that means your body is lying fallow 23 hours a day. We have become so removed from our natural movement patterns that our bodies are a mess. All that sitting has left our hips tight, our hamstrings and calves shortened, and our glutes weak. Our bodies have forgotten how to move the right way.

To reawaken our distant memories of correct movement, you'll have to relearn how to do one of the most natural activities: running.

Some people may recoil at that. *Learn* how to run—when we were *born* that way? Seems crazy, right? But the reality is that natural

Ultimately, it does not matter what type of running shoes you wear as long as you run using proper technique.

running in the modern era is an acquired skill, no different than a beginning golfer taking golf lessons, a tennis novice taking tennis lessons, a rookie guitar player taking guitar lessons.

As far as your corrupted-by-the-modern-world body is concerned, running the way that nature intended actually requires increased strength and new neurological patterns. If you want to run correctly and injury-free, you must drop the notion that because you ran as a kid—or even do a marathon a month now—you already know how to run—and don't need lessons. Wrong! You know about as much about running as a high school freshman does about throwing a javelin for the first time. He knows how to throw a stick, but it's not going to go very far without learning the specifics of good technique. But it isn't difficult. In fact, with a few simple cues and a basic understanding of physics, you can take advantage of the evolutionary gifts bestowed upon you to run efficiently and injury-free.

Those who have studied running techniques even briefly have most likely heard of the Chi Running, Pose, and barefoot running methods, which as a group share a bias against the heel strike—with which I don't disagree. People were not designed to land on their heels. The heel strike gives you a "braking" effect—that is, it slows you down—and a potential "breaking" effect—meaning that it transmits far too much shock up your leg and into your knee, hip, and spinal joints and can lead to injury.

Does this mean that I'm completely in sync with Chi, Pose, and barefoot advocates? Not necessarily. I think they tend to make running more complicated than it needs to be and don't fully understand how to exploit all of the built-in efficiencies of the human body. My approach to proper running technique focuses on what happens to the leg at the joints of the pelvis, hip, and knee, and where your foot hits the ground in reference to your center of gravity. When you use these joints properly, the foot strike takes care of itself.

The Three Big Changes

I can change a runner's gait for the better in 6 minutes. And you can, too. If you read this section and go out and practice these three specific changes, your gait and performance will improve immediately and you will spare yourself most of the common running injuries.

To develop a deeper understanding, continue reading past this section and delve into the physics involved. Time and time again at my Phase IV Scientific Health & Performance Center, a private training center with an exercise physiology lab attached that I opened in 2003 to bring science-based training to age-group athletes, we'll put runners on the treadmill, videotape their normal running style, and coach them into better mechanics. When they see their videotaped change in form, it never ceases to leave them astounded—especially because we've only asked them to do three relatively simple things:

- Adopt a vertical arm swing.

- Lift their knees a little higher.

- Speed up their cadence.

Here's why these three things work:

1. Adopt a vertical arm swing.

If you correct your arm swing, you'll balance your body, eliminate misdirected motion and excessive torque on joints, and run faster. *Every action creates a reaction* is a basic law of physics that holds true for your body when running. When something on the left side of the body moves, there has to be a counterbalancing movement on the right side in order to remain upright and balanced. The ideal counterbalance from a pure energy-cost point of view is one that will take the least amount of effort. So, when the right leg swings forward and the resulting forces want to rotate your trunk and shoulders to the left, you could flex the muscles of the midsection (your abs and lower back) to keep you in balance—but that has a high energy cost. The lowest energy cost would be to leave the midsection alone and simply swing your left arm straight forward to prevent your trunk from rotating. And the most economical way to swing the arm is like a pendulum.

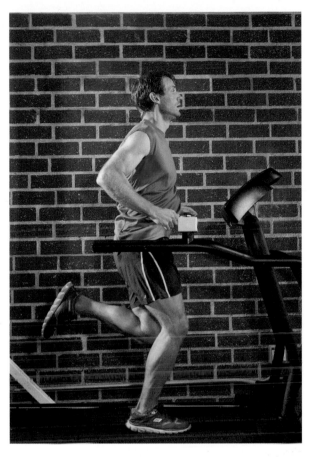

A good arm swing with arm bent slightly less than 90 degrees.

The arm should move like a pendulum anchored at the shoulder, with the weight of the hand acting to keep the pendulum swinging. To be most efficient, this pendulum arm swing must have two features: first, a vertical arc that does not angle crosswise over your chest. This arc directs all your effort to moving forward, eliminating the side-to-side body rotation that costs you a lot of energy, slows you down, and puts extra stress and wear on your joints. Second, the arm should have an ideal bend slightly more open

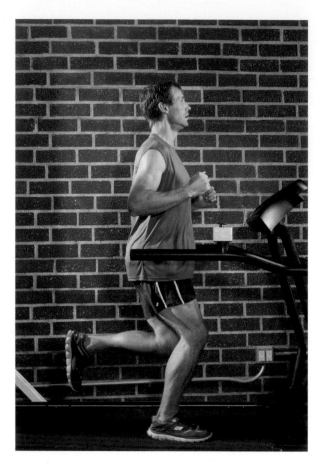

An example of bad form: arm swing with an excessive "Tyrannosaurus rex" elbow bend.

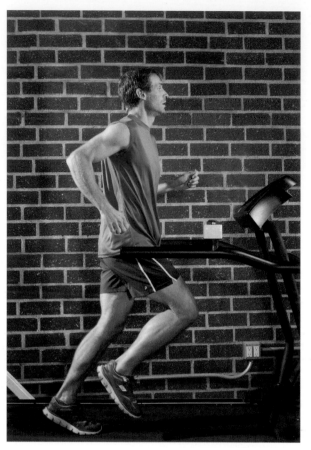

Good arm backswing with proper bend at the elbow.

than a 90-degree right angle. This bend allows the weight of the hand to swing the arm like a pendulum, which is more energy efficient than balancing the leg motion with the trunk muscles.

In helping the arm pendulum swing better, the backswing is often ignored. Although it might seem easy to push your elbows back a couple of inches behind the plane of your back (which then lets your arms easily swing forward), many people can't do it. That's because of tight pecs, which you get from too many push-ups

and bench presses and sitting scrunched up at a desk all day. Many runners are too tight to achieve adequate backswing, and this reduces the arm's tendency to move back and forth like a pendulum. So to develop a good backswing, we have to stretch the pectorals.

2. Lift your knees a little higher.

Most runners have inadequate front knee lift, which is usually because of weak hip flexors and core, and tight glutes and hamstrings. The

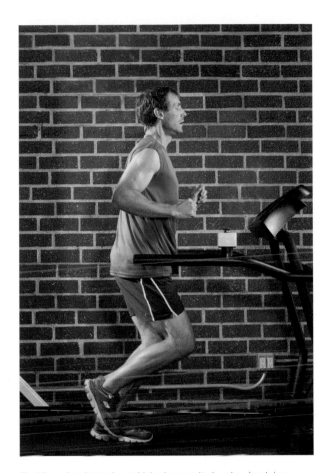

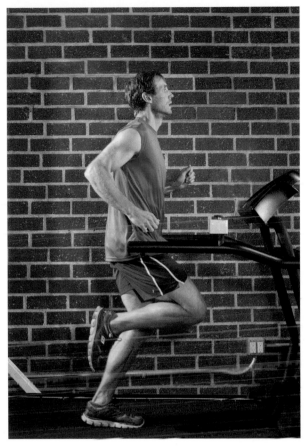

Bad form: low knee rise, which also results in a low heel rise in back and heel strike while the leg is still swinging forward.

Good form: high knee rise created by the hip flexing to at least 45 degrees, heel rises naturally toward the butt.

low lift penalizes them with the most common inefficiency in running: landing with the lower leg still swinging forward when it hits the ground, leading to a significant braking effect on their forward momentum.

To minimize this effect, the lower leg and foot must actually be moving backward when the foot strikes the ground. This is made possible by a high knee lift, accomplished by hip flexion of at least 40 to 50 degrees, which

gives the lower leg enough time to finish swinging forward and then begin moving backward before the foot strike. Technically, what's happening here is that the leg has enough height and time to swing, pendulum-like, back to the center while the elasticity of the hamstrings' and glutes' connective tissues snaps the leg back. The result: no braking effect—your foot is traveling backward as it lands below your center of gravity.

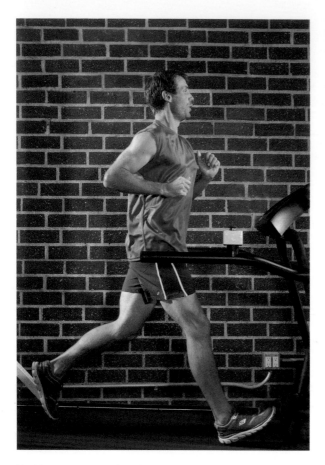

Bad form: bad heel strike in front of the body.

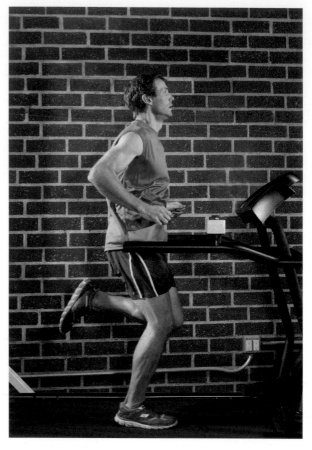

Good form: foot lands under the body, mid-foot striking first.

3. Speed up your cadence.

Long, slow strides thrust a straight leg out ahead of your body, making it impossible not to land on your heel or under your center of gravity. Every millimeter that your foot hits the ground in front of your center of gravity increases the braking effect on your forward momentum. The solution is simple: Increase your turnover. Run shorter strides with faster turnover. Because stride frequency and stride length are inversely related, the more steps you take per minute the shorter each step will be and the closer you will land beneath your center of gravity.

To be efficient, improve performance, and dramatically reduce your chance of getting injured, take 180 steps per minute (30 steps every 10 seconds), regardless of your speed. You'll benefit from increased cadence in several ways, whether you're a 10-minute miler or a 6-minute miler.

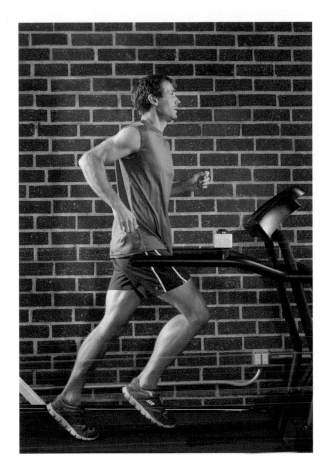

Bad form: lower leg moves forward before foot strike.

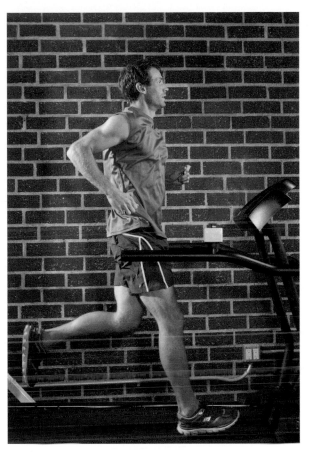

Good form: lower leg finishes the forward swing and begins to move backward before foot strike.

First, and most important, a fast cadence minimizes the braking effect, thereby reducing the overall energy required to maintain your pace. Second, shorter steps break up the workload into smaller chunks, which allow your muscles to make a less intense, more aerobic effort that keeps you in a greater fat-burning mode.

Be aware that the higher knee lift and faster cadence will seem harder at first. That's because that you, as a modern human, are starting in a weakened state. Initially, you won't have the strength to lift the knee high and turn your legs over swiftly. This is where the strength and flexibility exercises in chapters 7 and 8 come in. They will create your ability to exploit the built-in efficiency that nature intended.

STRIDE-CHANGING TRAINING DRILLS

The best way to work into this more efficient higher cadence running technique is to practice on a treadmill, which allows you to see the seconds go by and count your steps. Also, treadmill running is less taxing, because the ground is moving under you and all you have to do is really launch yourself in the air and then land, reducing the energy expenditure of running.

Begin with a 10-minute warm-up at your normal training pace. Without increasing the speed of the treadmill, practice a mix of your new faster/shorter and your old slower/longer strides. Start off with 2 minutes at a faster cadence, gradually building up to 30 steps every 10 seconds. Every foot strike, right and left, counts as one step. If you are like nearly every runner I have evaluated over the past 30 years, you will be taking about 25 or 26 steps per 10 seconds. The 4- or 5-step deficit does not seem like much of a problem, but it is. Per minute it adds up to 25 fewer steps, per mile it represents hundreds of inefficient steps, and thousands over the course of a 10k or longer.

At first, after 2 minutes of the faster cadence, you will be breathing harder and getting fatigued, so go back to your old lumbering gait and recover for 3 minutes. Repeat this for the duration of your workout and then build up to 3 minutes on/2 minutes off, and 4 on/1 off over the coming weeks. Soon, you'll have the strength to keep up the efficient high stride count and harvest the energy savings of running with the laws of physics, instead of fighting them. In addition to working on a faster cadence, there are four drills that will facilitate proper running mechanics: arm swing, high knee, butt kick, and Cossack, described in "Running Mechanics Drills" on pages 34–35. Do 2 reps of these drills each for 30 seconds after you have warmed up, twice per week.

Running with the Laws of Physics

To fully understand the whys of proper running mechanics and how to use your body correctly when running, we have to talk a little about a few simple laws of physics:

MOMENTUM

A body in motion tends to stay in motion unless some force acts to impede its progress. Every time your foot hits the ground, the foot-ground reaction acts to slow you down. Every millimeter that your foot strikes the ground in front of your center of gravity further increases the braking effect on your forward momentum. The center of gravity of your body is the center of your weight distribution, the point where your body would teeter on a focal point if you were lying horizontal in space. This spot is located in the back of the pelvis. Left to our own devices, all of us *overstride*—that is, land way too far in front of a line dropped from the center of gravity to the ground below us. This not only wastes energy as we try to regain forward momentum, but it causes us to land on the heel of the outstretched leg and leads to injury from the excessive shock forces. So when it comes to foot strike, it is not which part of your foot hits the ground first, it's where your foot hits the ground in relationship to your center of gravity that will either minimize ground reaction or amplify it—that is, either slow you down or let you move forward more easily with less effort. A higher knee rise and shorter steps ensure that your foot will hit the ground more directly under your hips.

SLINGS AND SPRINGS

The human body is made of sinewy connective tissues that stretch under the load of our body weight when we hit the ground. The stretched tissues store what is called *potential energy*; just like a rubber band that snaps back to its original form, the rebounding tendons, ligaments, and fascia give back that stored energy and provide much of the forces needed to propel us forward. If we use our body in the right way, these rebounding tissues can unburden the muscles of some of the work and save energy, allowing you to run farther and faster. You harness this elastic energy by keeping your connective tissues flexible and running with high knees to keep the leg swinging backward when it hits the ground.

PENDULUMS

A pendulum is a line, weighted at the bottom, which swings in an arc from a fixed anchor point above. It requires very little energy at the beginning of the movement to stay in motion. The most efficient way for the extremities to swing through the air is for them to act like pendulums. Pendulums require gravity to keep them moving because when they swing forward, they hold stored potential energy because gravity wants to swing them back to the bottom of the arc. With little muscular energy at the start of the arm and leg swing, your extremities will return to their place of origin and save muscle energy.

Using a high knee in running serves several purposes. First, it allows us the time needed to be sure the pendulum has finished its forward swing and is moving backward when your foot hits the ground. Second, a high knee rise automatically brings your heel closer to your butt and shortens the length of the pendulum that is your leg. Shortening the swinging lever reduces the energy needed to swing it through the air and therefore reduces the work your hip flexors need to do to pull your leg forward. Last, a high knee rise and the lower leg naturally pulled up closer to your butt reduces wind resistance. It is not only beneficial when there is a headwind, but even on a calm day your body has to push itself through the standing air, and this energy savings adds up over longer distances.

RUNNING MECHANICS DRILLS

After doing a full set of the runners' stretches in chapter 7 (pages 120–138), and completing a 15-minute warmup run, perform each of these drills for 10 to 20 meters (33 to 67 feet) and repeat 2 to 4 times with a minute rest between repetitions. Do the drills once the first week and then twice a week. Do not work through pain.

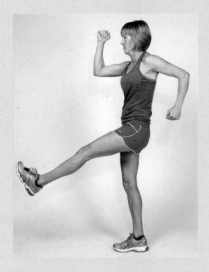 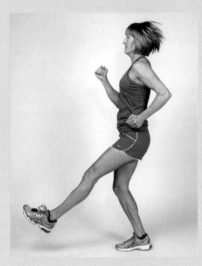 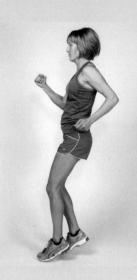

COSSACK DANCE DRILL

This exercise activates the glutes and upper hamstrings to pull your leg back under your pelvis before your foot hits the ground.

1. Start with a good arm swing.

2. Keep an upright posture and hold your legs straight. Kick your leg forward and then snap it back to land under your pelvis.

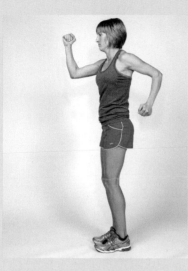 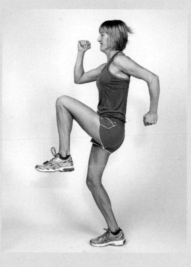 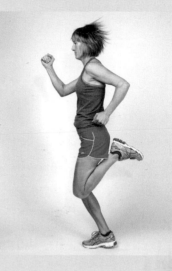

ARM DRILLS

Proper arm swing opens the torso to improve breathing and facilitate high knee lift on the opposite side.

1. Stand in place with elbows flexed at 90 degrees and chest up.

2. Move your arms forward and backward like a pendulum hinging from the shoulders, with your elbows staying at the same angle throughout the vertical arm swing. Note: Don't allow your arms to swing across your torso and limit your trunk rotation.

HIGH KNEE LIFTS

Proper knee lift sets up for the proper foot strike directly below the pelvis.

1. Start with a good arm swing.

2. Begin marching, lifting your knees so that your thighs are almost parallel to the ground. Move forward at a moderate pace.

3. Work to land each step softly near your mid-foot.

BUTT KICKS

Butt kicks facilitate the high back heel rise that comes with good mechanics.

1. Start with a good arm swing.

2. Run forward without much speed, holding your knees straight down below your pelvis. Kick your heel back toward your butt, but don't force the movement.

WHAT IS OVERPRONATION?

If someone tells you that you are a pronator, say thank you. Foot pronation is the first of a series of natural events that occurs in the joints of your legs and pelvis to achieve shock absorption. Overpronation, however, does the opposite. It reduces the shock absorption capabilities of your body. If you are identified as an overpronator, before changing to motion control shoes or getting fit for custom orthotic devices, you need to first correct your mechanics. This correction will not only help prevent injury, but improve efficiency. To understand why, here's an explanation of how good running form absorbs shock and how overpronation differs from normal pronation.

When the foot hits the ground, it sets off a sequence of shock-absorbing events that starts with the collapse of your arch and moves up through your leg, knee, hip, and pelvis. Acting as nature's own shock absorbers, your joints, muscles, tendons, and fascia work in harmony to absorb forces up to three times your body weight and lower your center of gravity with great energy efficiency.

Once the arch collapses into pronation and unlocks the joints of the midfoot, the foot is transformed into a flexible posture better able to adapt to the terrain. The foot pronation causes the shin bone to rotate inwardly, which bends the knee and also allows the hip to flex. By midstance, the center of gravity has efficiently descended to its lowest point in the gait cycle.

At midstance, the foot should be fully pronated. As the opposite leg swings through and brings the pelvis forward, this causes the weight-bearing side of the pelvis to rotate backward and unwind the inward rotation of the thigh and shin bone that occurred in the pronation cycle. As the weight-bearing thigh and shin are rotated back outward, this pulls the weight-bearing foot out of its flexible pronated position into a rigid supinated posture that provides a rigid foot to push off. This is the most energy-efficient way to transport a runner's center of gravity from point A to point B.

The overpronator is someone who, for reasons having to do with variations in foot anatomy, continues to pronate past midstance. If the weight-bearing leg is still torqued in a pronated stance as the opposite leg swings through, when the foot should be starting to resupinate to provide a rigid lever to push off, it is still pronated and flexible. This causes the runner to push off on a flexible pronated foot; that is energy inefficient, because the muscles of the leg and foot now must work extra hard to stabilize a foot that should already be locked and rigid in supination. This makes the weight-bearing leg vulnerable to excessive forces that, over time, will cause tissue breakdown and injury.

The best prevention and treatment for injuries related to overpronation is accomplished by correcting the runner's gait. The high knee and faster cadence of good running form reduces the contact time between the foot and ground and limits the degree of overpronation by limiting the time the foot has to deviate from normal mechanics. The lesson, taught for decades by elite coaches I've worked with, never changes: Fix the mechanics and the injuries will disappear.

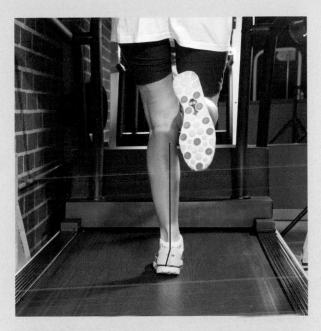

Overpronation from posterior: see divergent angle of the heel and lower leg.

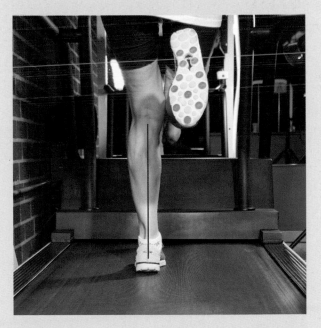

Pronation corrected with higher cadence: see the heel aligned with the lower leg.

Shoes: Form Trumps Cushioning

I am no advocate of barefoot running, which in practice can cause far too many injuries, especially to foot bones, Achilles tendons, and calves not used to the new biomechanics. That, and the basic lack of protection for the bottom of the foot, is why the enthusiasm for barefooting faded away after the book *Born to Run* gave it a brief boost starting in 2009. So you have to wear shoes. But what kind? Shoes aren't perfect, either, because many were designed imperfectly from the start and built on the premise that overstriding is normal.

The shoe companies chased the natural tendency of untrained runners to overstride and heel strike, and actually made it worse. The big, clunky pillow of heel cushioning that has progressed in size over the years to accommodate bad form gets in the way of you pulling your leg backward to land under your center of gravity and prevents you from landing more toward your

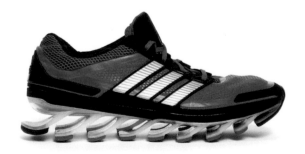

Large clunky heel

midfoot. This design makes it harder to clear the ground when you try to pull your foot back. The giant heel pads and the rear-shoe rise that go with it are unnecessary and unwieldy.

Does this mean I advocate flat, low-profile "minimalist" shoes? Well, despite not being a fan of the superskimpy ones, I ultimately think it does not matter what shoes you wear, as long as you run correctly. Runners who run with good mechanics don't need artificial shock absorption between the ground and their feet, because the natural "slings and springs" of good technique will take care of that. With good technique, your joints perform the shock absorption. A firm sole and adequate heel counter is all most people need for protection, because the reduced ground contact of the faster cadence means you're not on the ground long enough to overpronate (see "What Is Overpronation?" on pages 36–37), thereby cutting the risk of injuries.

That said, we're tender-footers. As mentioned previously, I see a host of maladies resulting from going barefoot or wearing minimalist shoes, including plantar fasciitis, bone bruises, stress fractures, and strained tendons.

There are two groups that, even after fixing their running technique, often still have a tendency to experience injuries: Extreme overpronators and heavy people (which can include overweight people or anyone, even very fit, weighing more than 200 pounds [90.7 kg]). If

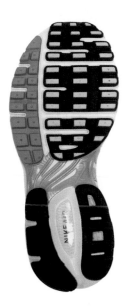

Sole of motion control shoe with mid-foot stabilization arch

SUMMARY

To prevent injuries and increase speed, runners must eliminate the heel strike and the overstriding that causes it. Humans, hindered by bodies weakened by modern life and thickly cushioned running shoes, can reestablish their old movement patterns by focusing on three areas: the vertical arm swing, high knee raise, and rapid cadence of 180 steps per minute.

their problems persist, they need bona fide motion control shoes.

Overpronators need shoes with more stability, especially in the form of a rigid heel cup to keep the heel from flopping inward at foot strike. Because overpronation is an energy suck, as you are pushing off from an unstable foot instead of a stable one, motion control shoes will also make their wearers faster.

By the same token, heavy folks just need more shoe—with a denser midsole and heel counter, usually a motion control shoe—because they pound the ground with more force due to their bulk. Whereas a lighter person can mostly rely on technique to absorb shock and let the shoe do the rest in a 70:30 ratio, that ratio will be more like 50:50 for a heavy person.

3 The Science of Recovery

Recovery, which is the foundation of the Four Pillars in the House of Health and Performance, is the missing link of training. Do it and your health and performance improve. Don't do it and you risk a host of overtraining problems such as sickness, injuries, a bad attitude, and poor results.

You're feeling a little lethargic. Unmotivated. Fatigued. Sometimes you're tired enough to fall asleep at the drop of a hat, yet unable to sleep after you wake up in the middle of the night. True, you've lost weight, added muscle, and increased speed because of your workouts—but lately you've been a little apathetic, not looking forward to them, maybe even starting to get more colds and injuries here and there. So what's the problem—aren't you doing the work?

Well, maybe the problem is that you're doing *too much* work—or too much of the same work. Either way, you are *overtrained*, and why that has happened is because you are probably shorting yourself on *recovery*.

Recovery is the great missing link in most training plans. Eastern European training guru Tudor Bompa famously said, "Recovery should be so well understood and actively enhanced that it becomes a fixed component of your training." That's because recovery is the crucial low-intensity time that your body needs to heal and rebuild itself so that it comes back stronger, more efficient than before. On the macro level, recovery includes taking it easy the days after hard workouts and taking one day off altogether every week; on the micro level, it includes paying more attention to your cooldown, stretching, and post-workout nutrition and hydration. Honor the recovery day—it's when the benefits of your hard training are realized.

There are several ways that you can short yourself on recovery and become overtrained. You might have rushed your base training so your body is overstressed from a too-compressed Periodization schedule that didn't give it time to gradually adapt. Or maybe you haven't varied your training stimulus, week after week doing the same semi-hard runs, the same distance, the same hills, so not only is your body getting stale and not improving, it is always functioning with a low level of fatigue from lack of rest.

Your workouts become less productive because fatigued muscles start each workout underfueled (that is, short on glycogen, which is what carbohydrates become when stored in the muscles and liver for use as energy). Thus, you can't produce the intensity needed in your next workout to build your fitness, yet you are not going easy enough to allow for recovery. In this manner, all your workouts become skewed to mediocrity—never going easy enough to recover and not having the energy to work hard enough to improve. Also, when you train with chronic fatigue from going too hard all the time, you cannot maintain proper running mechanics, and as mechanics break down, the risk of injury increases.

Additionally, an underrecovered body builds up too much cortisol, which is a stress hormone that makes your body store fat and water and slows down your metabolism—the opposite of your training goals. In short, depriving yourself of recovery means that you're doing all the work but getting rewarded with poor results, injuries, and sickness.

"Working hard is easy—everyone knows how to work hard. But those who know how to work hard at recovery are the ones who win," says my friend and mentor, coach Bob Kersee, the most successful track and field coach of all time. Fact: Athletes by nature know how to push it, but the ones who know when to throttle back perform the best. Therefore, to make sure you recover, don't leave it to chance. Program recovery into your workout schedule and rigorously observe it.

The Big Three Recovery Killers

Overtraining syndrome and lack of recovery are two sides of the same coin, and unfortunately, the rule rather than the exception. Avoid them by guarding against slipping into these three bad training habits:

- **Falling into a Rut.** Beware of doing the same thing, such as running your standard 6-mile (9.6-km) loop, every day, over and over. Your body adapts to the stress of a particular workout to the point where it is hardly stressful anymore. As a result, your workouts will no longer elicit a strong hormonal response. Instead, your hormones just say "ho-hum" and fade. To keep improving, you need to keep changing the stress every 8 weeks per the Periodization schedule outlined in chapter 4.

- **Doing Too Much Too Soon.** Although your breathing and organs—heart and lungs—adapt rapidly to the stress of increased exercise, your infrastructure—bones, joints, and muscles—do not. So you need the discipline to keep from going as fast as your breathing will let you; otherwise, your body's infrastructure won't be able to deal with the stress. In Periodization terms, you don't want to rush the base-building phase. Don't do any hard workouts—such as intervals or hills—on a too-shallow base.

- **Going Too Hard All the Time.** Some people never stop, never give themselves recovery time, and it eventually comes back to hurt them. Too much intensity—hard running, biking, skiing, you name it, sometimes on the same day—will negatively impact your health. Do not violate the hard-easy paradigm of Periodization.

The Ten Commandments of Recovery and Preventing Overtraining

To understand the importance of recovery, the risks of overtraining, and the strategy for getting the most out of your training, approach recovery as a science. Do it by following these ten steps:

1. Remember the Supercompensation Principle of Progressive Overload.

The foundation of all successful training is *supercompensation*, a principle in which increasing stress triggers an adaptive response that strengthens the body's physiological systems. Following hard work, you at first feel fatigued and suffer an initial decrease in performance; then, with recovery, the body becomes stronger and more efficient. We can't overemphasize the point that these improvements occur only if time for recovery is provided.

Periodization training is a stepchild of recovery, born out of the need to avoid mental and physical burnout and achieve peak performance when it counts most. A well-designed Periodization program manipulates intensity (how hard you train and the volume, i.e., the total number of miles or hours you train each week), manipulating them to create the right amount of stress on the body.

As mentioned, endurance athletes' big problem often is that their structural system (foundational infrastructure such as tendons, bone, and fascia) can't handle the high training load necessary to take them to their peak. Additionally, the metabolic system can be overtaxed and weakened with an inappropriate balance of stress and recovery.

2. Honor Your Base Training.

Remember that low-intensity, early-season base training is when you build your metabolic and structural foundation that will support the harder training efforts later in the season. A good example is vascularization, which is essentially the increased formation of blood vessels. Improved vascularization is only stimulated by low-intensity workouts and aids recovery by ensuring the presence of blood vessels close to each working muscle cell, thereby providing a quick exchange of waste products and oxygen and nutrients with the muscles.

Other examples of foundational structures enhanced by base building include your skeleton, joints, and muscles, all of which help maintain form and economy of motion as you run, translating to fewer injuries and easier, faster recovery. It's the same story with the enhanced fat-burning metabolism you develop during base training; a lower production of lactic acid and waste products along with a lessened reliance on carbohydrates as fuel makes bonking, or hitting a wall, and cannibalizing muscle less likely, again allowing for a faster recovery.

Need I say it again? Better recovery today translates to the ability to work harder tomorrow.

3. Alternate Hard and Easy Workouts and Build in Rest Periods. Use Light Workouts for an Active Recovery.

A hard workout can be a long workout or a high-intensity workout; it stimulates the adaptations that make you stronger, but those gains actually occur on the easy, active-recovery day that follows. Similarly, your training program must have built-in recovery weeks following every 2 to 3 weeks of building intensity. At the end of your yearly training cycle, you need 3 to 6 weeks of chill time to allow complete system recovery.

Active recovery is better than rest alone. There is nothing passive about recovery. Yes, you can get some recovery by sitting on the couch and eating Cheetos the day after a hard workout. But the best recovery is an active process in which light "adaptation" workouts, such as an easy-paced run, swim, bicycle ride, or even walk, stimulate recovery better than rest alone. Light workouts are akin to the self-cleaning oven, in which the heat is turned up but no roast is placed inside. They provide the body the same opportunity to do housecleaning functions without having to recover from the damaging effects of a new workout. Light exercise increases circulation, releases testosterone and other recovery hormones, and activates "heat shock" proteins in the body to repair damaged muscles and tissues. These processes are only set in place when you heat up the body from the inside out with light exercise (sorry, hot tubs don't work because external heat only increases inflammation instead of decreasing it). Similar occurrences improve connective tissue and bone repair as well. The danger is letting the active recovery workout become too strenuous.

4. Perception of Fatigue Is Not Reality.

The fact is that most people can't objectively view themselves and their training, and don't realize which levels of fatigue are okay and which are debilitating. The likelihood of uncoached athletes becoming overtrained is high because they will increase their training load when they "perceive" a plateau or decrease in

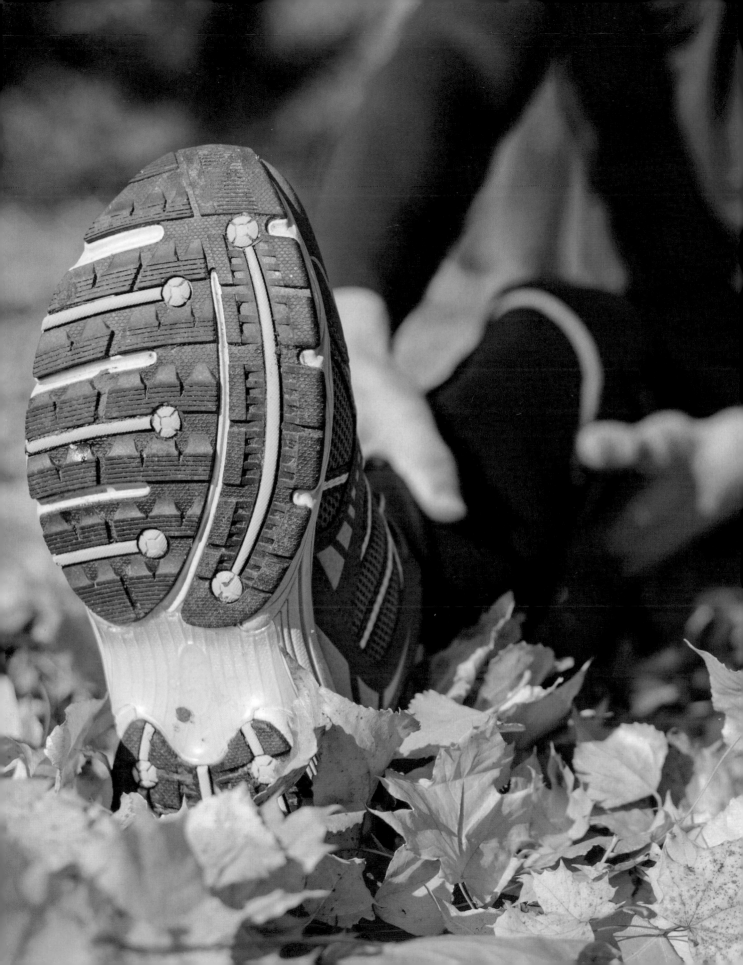

performance—which, in many cases, is exactly what they shouldn't do. A well-designed program accounts for the fatigue and performance deficits associated with hard training, then provides the recovery time you need for supercompensation to kick in. So don't wing it. Train by science, not by whim. A safe, effective training schedule takes the guesswork out of recovery by including regular days and weeks of rest and recovery, insulating you from the natural tendency to overdo it.

5. Change Your Training after 8 Weeks.

A cornerstone of recovery and Periodization training as a whole is a meaningful variation in training stimulus, which keeps the body and mind fresh. The body, driven by hormones, is designed to adapt quickly to exercise; in fact, after about 8 weeks of a certain type of exercise, you achieve full adaptation, meaning you've improved about as much as possible with that particular training stimulus. So, to facilitate further growth, you have to alter the exercise stress. This keeps the body constantly off balance and forces further adaptation with another hormonal release to avoid staleness.

Variety also furthers what you might call "mental recovery"—helping you keep focus and motivation high and avoiding mental burnout.

6. Stretch before and after Every Workout.

Stretching before workouts improves your mechanics and reduces wear and tear on your muscles, tendons, and joints. After workouts, stretching wrings the waste products, such as lactic acid, out of the muscles and returns muscles to their normal resting length, avoiding muscle and tendon shortening. In this way, your stretching efforts go further toward elongating connective tissue and helping tendons and ligaments heal and grow stronger. A good indication of when your structural system is recovered and ready for another hard workout is when the stiffness from the most recent hard workout is absent.

Stretching provides the body the range of motion that is required around the joints for the correct running biomechanics and minimizes the damage created during workouts. Workouts are far more productive when unencumbered by the tightness that would otherwise occur following hard exercise.

Static stretching exercises, in which you hold a position while motionless, are the best for zapping stiffness and elongating tissues. Don't rely on a "dynamic" warm-up (a new trend that involves active range-of-motion movements, as opposed to static stretching) or a slow jog to start your workout. Although these can be part of your warm-up, they are not substitutes for static stretching.

7. Perform Self-Massage before and after Every Workout.

Self-massage and using a foam roller (a simple, condensed-foam cylinder 4 or 5 inches [10 or 12.5 cm] in diameter that you lie upon with your body weight) are excellent methods to aid recovery, preferably after workouts, but any time of the day will do. Both manipulate the muscles and tissue, which increases blood flow, breaks adhesions, and promotes adaptation of connective tissue. No specific knowledge or training is necessary. For self-massage, just take some lotion and begin rubbing your calf and thigh muscles, front and back. With the roller, hit the long muscles in your legs from bottom to top. You will feel the fatigue and tension leave your body. (See the foam roller workout on pages 172–173.)

8. Ice Sore and Tight Areas.

Ice reduces inflammation, muscle tightness, and spasm, and allows muscles to relax and recover better. Ice helps avoid injuries and treats minor irritations before they develop into overuse syndromes.

Ice isn't just for injuries—it is essential to all of your recovery efforts. By controlling runaway inflammation, it helps your body adapt in more functional ways to the stress of your workouts. Although inflammation is the first essential step in the body's structural repair and improvement process, science has shown that it can be excessive; by overriding it with icing, we speed up recovery, enabling you to work hard again sooner. Ice helps avoid injuries and treats minor irritations (microtrauma) before they develop into overuse syndromes (macrotrauma). Icing and ice baths reduce levels of cortisol, the stress hormone that stalls your metabolic recovery.

Put ice cubes and water in a plastic, zippered bag or commercial bag with rubber on the inside and cloth covering outside and apply to tight and sore areas for 20 minutes once or twice a day to relieve tightness or soreness. Gel packs are not as effective.

9. Use Compression Clothing to Squeeze the Waste Products Out of Your Muscles.

Compression garments act like a massage, flushing the waste products and swelling out of your muscles after workouts. Lower-extremity tights are built to create a funnel-like compression force that is greatest at the ankle and calf and lessens through the thighs to empty the vascular capillary beds where blood pools after workouts. Put them on directly after your workouts or after you shower and then perform your post-workout stretching and foam roller routine. You can ice right through them or even wear them in an ice bath to maximize your recovery efforts. They combat the subtle swelling of the ankles and legs that results from elevated levels of the stress hormone cortisol.

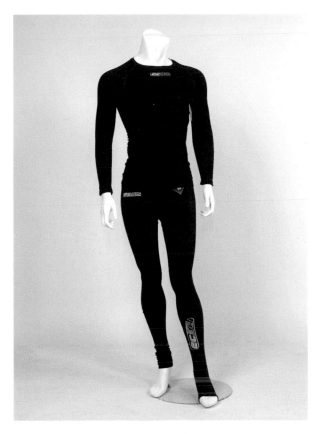

Compression top and tights

muscles to absorb carbs and protein.) Fruit and any sweets will do except for chocolate, which has too much fat, slowing the rate at which the carbs will leave your stomach and arrive at your depleted muscles. Furthermore, research shows that food or drink with a 4-to-1 mixture of carbs to protein (a ratio pioneered by Endurox, made by Pacific Health Labs, which we've success-fully tested on our athletes) stimulates a larger insulin reaction and speeds recovery. Within an hour, follow up with a balanced meal of carbs, protein, and fat. Then continue to graze until you feel satiated. In this way, you can reach full glycogen recovery within 4 hours, whereas if you missed the 15-minute window, it can take up to 24 hours to restore glycogen levels in the liver and muscles.

Back-to-back long or difficult workouts can create a constant glycogen-depleted state, which hampers muscle function and leads to a breakdown in running mechanics and produces more stress and injuries.

10. Take Advantage of the 15-Minute Nutrition Window.

Get food and drink into your body within 15 minutes of your workout. This "window" is when your body is most susceptible to receiving nu-trients. Circulation is high, making delivery from your gut to your muscles easy.

This is the time to feed your sweet tooth with high-glycemic (sugary) carbohydrates to begin rebuilding your glycogen stores. (Tech-nically, the sugary stuff releases insulin from your pancreas, which opens the windows in the

WATER WORKOUTS WORK WONDERS

In 1987, just 3 weeks before the Track and Field World Championships in Rome, Italy, Florence "Flo-Jo" Griffith went down with a grade II hamstring strain. Grade II is not as bad as a full-blown muscle tear (that's grade III), but it's bad enough to destroy your hopes in an event that close and set you back for months, especially if you're a world-class athlete. Florence was limping, suffering swelling and sudden flashes of pain, and experiencing deep pain when I pressed in on the hamstring muscle and tried to bend her knee against resistance.

Yet she ended up doing great at the Worlds. That's because we used water running, a remarkably valuable recovery tool that all runners—injured or not—should take advantage of.

Combining flotation with hydrostatic pressure, running in the water gives you a nearly impact-free workout with six times the resistance you experience while moving through the air; that allows you to rehab and strengthen still-healing body parts while maintaining fitness and form.

In Flo-Jo's case, we had to act fast to fix her hamstring, maintain fitness, and keep her confidence up for the Worlds, a key pre-Olympic event. This wouldn't be easy. Athletes like her are finely tuned machines, and removing her from the track and missing the all-important tapering and peaking phase of training would normally leave her at a subpar level.

So I proceeded with the PRICE protocol for acute injuries. After we got inflammation under control with ice, ultrasound, and electric stimulation, I began administering cross-fiber friction massage to break up dysfunctional scar tissue that formed in the injured muscle. Once Florence could walk without pain, I supported her thigh with a self-grip compression wrap and got her in the pool at my clinic in Santa Monica. At first, because it even hurt for her to perform the running motion in the water, I had her do a "wooden soldier" water walking exercise, in which she imitated walking like a wooden soldier with straight arms and legs while she was held afloat by a foam device around her waist. This workout is harder than water running because of the drag created by the increased surface area of the outstretched extremities.

After a few more days of two-a-day physical therapy treatments, Florence was able to run in the water without pain, so we began matching her workouts in the water to the workouts her teammates were doing on that track. If Coach Kersee called for the other 200-meter sprinters on his team to do 3 x 400 meters at a 53-second pace with a rest interval of 1 minute, and then 3 x 200 meters at a 23-second pace with 30 seconds of rest, we did the same times in the pool. We matched workout for workout with the team.

Within 2 weeks, Florence was ready to return part-time to the track. After 1 week of workouts on the UCLA track, augmented by more pool workouts at my office, we traveled to Italy and continued treatments to restore full strength and flexibility and clear up the last bit of scar tissue.

At the Worlds, Florence not only ran three heats of the 200-meter dash and the final without pain, but won the silver medal with a personal record of 21.96 (losing to East German sprint stalwart Silke Gladisch). But she wasn't done yet! Two days and lots of massages later, she ran a leg of the U.S. women's gold-medal-winning 4 x 100 meter relay.

If you're scratching your head over this, join the crowd. Two weeks of missed workouts on the track after suffering an injury that can end a sprinter's career and Florence runs her best time ever on her way to the silver medal and a gold medal? And she outperformed most of her teammates, too. How could this happen?

Well, I like to think my physical therapy techniques helped speed the healing of her injury, but the water was the key. Why? Probably a bit overtrained by a young coach Kersee, Florence's forced time off and the restorative benefits of the water workouts helped her recover a bit more

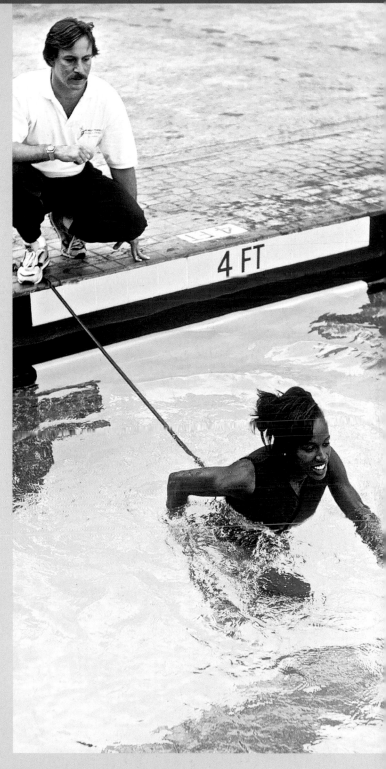

Robert Forster working with Olympic champion Jackie Joyner-Kersee doing a water workout.

than the others and peak when it counted. To be fair, her teammate Jackie Joyner-Kersee won double gold in both the heptathlon and the long jump events, soundly beating the Russians and Germans. But Jackie was in my office three times per week for recovery massage and preventive treatments even when she wasn't injured. In fact, the frequency of visits to my office for restorative therapies correlates exactly with the number of Olympic medals won by any individual on our team. Jackie came into the office the most and won the most medals (six); Florence was next in number of visits and she won five; and Gail Devers was third in the number of visits and won three Olympic gold medals.

After 1987, water workouts (which I ended up cowriting a book about, *The Complete Water-power Workout Book*) became a fixed component of our training and rehabilitation programs for all our clients. We found that runners can exploit the hydrostatic pressure that water exerts on their submerged bodies to facilitate recovery during low impact water workouts, or they can do high-powered intervals in the pool to gain the benefits and not the wear and tear. Also, because the water provides six times the resistance that your extremities encounter moving through the air, water workouts strengthen the hip flexors, core, and glutes to facilitate better mechanics and efficiency. The pool is a great environment for plyometric power workouts too, because the soft landings spare the joints from the otherwise extreme stress of these power moves when done on land. This is key for older runners who miss the benefits from the bounding and jumping work done in plyometric training because their joints can't take the pounding.

So, you know that pool in your backyard or at the gym that you never use because you don't like swimming? It's a key to happiness for all runners.

4 Periodization Training

To run a race to the best of your ability, and to do it with the least amount of injury, fatigue, and worry, nothing beats Periodization, a near-foolproof stair-step training plan that ramps you up safely and leaves you primed to fly.

If you just want to stay active and don't care about getting faster or losing large chunks of time to nagging injuries, keep doing your regular run. But if you want to improve, get fitter, stop getting injured, and maybe score a personal record at a race, your run-of-the-mill haphazard training won't cut it. To kick your running up several notches, you have to train in a way that is good for your body, building it up and speeding it up while limiting the potential for injuries.

To do that, you need a strategy that is almost bipolar, in that it combines increasingly hard efforts with rest days and rest weeks. Over the weeks and months, this hard-easy schedule is the paradigm that gives your body time to heal, recover, and build bigger, stronger, faster muscles and connective tissue.

Sequence is the key. The science shows that you have to properly sequence your training to develop one aspect of fitness at a time and then use that as a foundation to build the next. In fact, to be your fittest by the time the starting gun goes off, you must be incredibly patient. You will spend a long time building a broad base of aerobic infrastructure and musculoskeletal resiliency before adding on layers of higher-intensity work such as hill training and intervals as you approach race day. This strategy is virtually foolproof, used by the world's best athletes in every sport, and it'll work for you if you have the discipline to follow it.

It's called Periodization.

The foundation of all modern training, Periodization was officially christened in 1963 by Tudor Bompa, a former Olympic rower and faculty member of the Romanian Institute of Sport who trained eleven Olympic and World Championship medalists in track and field and rowing. But Soviet sports scientists had already been working on this type of training since the 1950s,

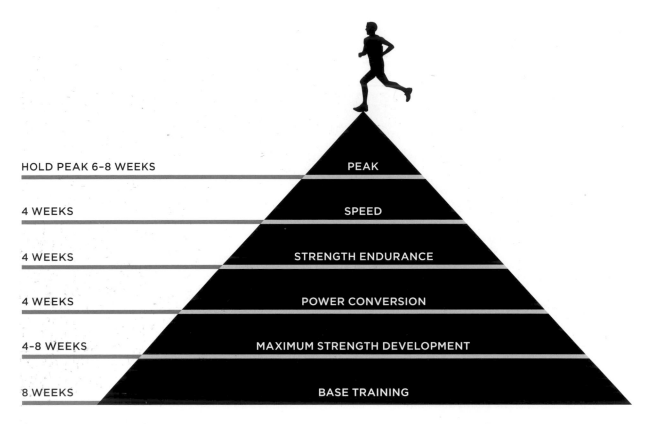

PHASES OF PERIODIZATION FITNESS PROGRESSION

HOLD PEAK 6–8 WEEKS	PEAK
4 WEEKS	SPEED
4 WEEKS	STRENGTH ENDURANCE
4 WEEKS	POWER CONVERSION
4–8 WEEKS	MAXIMUM STRENGTH DEVELOPMENT
8 WEEKS	BASE TRAINING

The volume of work is greatest in base training and must decrease with the higher intensity in successive Perodization training phases.

conducting controlled research on promising young athletes in isolated training facilities. Able to control diet, sleep, and environment while ignoring inconvenient Western concepts such as consent, they manipulated exercise stimulus in search of the most effective training program design. The results may have been ethically corrupt, but they proved to be scientifically sound.

What emerged was a model of human adaptation that provides predictable outcomes when exercise is orchestrated in a scientifically rational sequence. Of course, after what became known as Periodization was used with great success by Iron Curtain athletes, the West started getting on board with it in the 1970s.

Basically, the Periodization model builds the athlete up to optimal performance with a stair-step series of methodical, progressive challenges and recoveries that strengthen your body and keep brain and brawn fresh. It starts with a goal (such as a marathon or 10k) and plans a workout schedule leading up to it, breaking up your

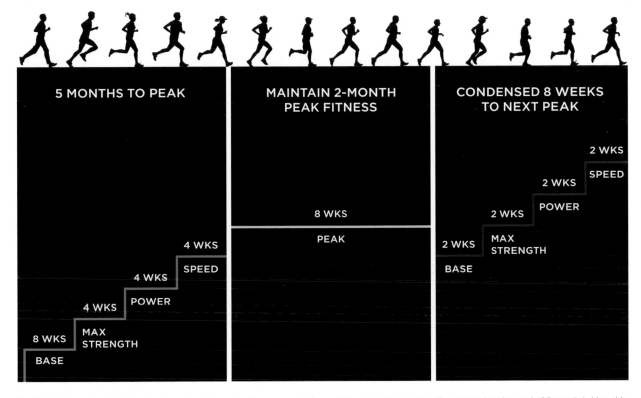

BI-PEAK YEARLY TRAINING PLAN

5 MONTHS TO PEAK

4 WKS — SPEED
4 WKS — POWER
4 WKS — MAX STRENGTH
8 WKS — MAX STRENGTH
BASE

MAINTAIN 2-MONTH PEAK FITNESS

8 WKS
PEAK

CONDENSED 8 WEEKS TO NEXT PEAK

2 WKS — SPEED
2 WKS — POWER
2 WKS — MAX STRENGTH
2 WKS — MAX STRENGTH
BASE

Periodization schedule showing how to achieve two fitness peaks (one at the end of 5 months, the second at the end of 8 weeks). Use this schedule when training for two races in one year, for example.

training time for your targeted event into five training cycles or phases, each with a specific fitness goal in mind.

Periodization plays out like this:

Phase 1: Base Training

This is an 8-week training cycle of gradually ramping up the miles, with the dual goal of building up your metabolic (oxygen-processing capacity) and structural foundation (bone, muscle, and joint strength) as well as your fueling system. The latter refers to using low-intensity "aerobic" training to teach your body to rely mainly on fat, which all bodies have a huge supply of, for fuel. The gradual ramp-up also hardens the structural components of your body against injury for the tougher workouts to come. At the same time, you also will be using light weights to build a strength base; that will isolate and strengthen all the little "helper" muscles that act to stabilize each joint and perfect your running mechanics.

Phase 2: Strength Development

This is a 4- to 8-week training cycle of gradually increasing intensity that uses hill running and weight lifting with heavy weights to increase the strength of the tendons, bones, and the bigger muscles that propel you forward.

Phase 3: Power Conversion

This is a 4-week training cycle designed to convert the strength developed in Phase 2 into running power—so that muscles can contract faster and harder. To do this, you need more anaerobic power, which is achieved with hill repeats and intervals and explosive movements in the gym with lighter-weight loads.

Phase 4: Speed or Strength Endurance

This is a 4-week cycle that brings your fitness to a peak of speed or strength endurance, depending on whether you are preparing for a 5k or 10k or the longer races. It uses shorter, harder intervals to hone your anaerobic fitness and super-lightweight loads in the gym for high-rep sets that make your muscles more fatigue resistant.

Phase 5: Taper and Peak

In this short period, usually the last 2 to 3 weeks before your event, you shorten your workouts but keep up the intensity, leaving you razor sharp and well rested to do your best on game day.

Phase 6: Transition

When it's over, you chill out a bit with easy running and cross-training designed for recovery. Then get ready to start all over again on the next goal by starting with base training again.

In a nutshell, Periodization proves that the development of substantial physiological infrastructure must precede the hard work of the later phases as you approach competition. Without developing the necessary infrastructure first through base training, and progressively in the strength development phase, the hard work needed to prepare for competition will not be as effective and also may not be tolerated, leading to injury, overtraining, or illness. Periodization's five training phases ultimately help you avoid the danger zone for all runners: overtraining, which leaves you burned out, sick, injured, and with suboptimal performances.

The Basic Laws of Periodization

Periodization Law #1: Recovery Is Essential

The most important thing to remember is that all work is futile if you don't allow recovery. No one ever became stronger during a workout; it's only afterward, during the recovery time, when your fitness evolves. Recovery is built into all Periodization training models because it's needed, whether you feel like you need it or not. Each week has hard and easy days of training, and every 4 weeks a lighter week is provided for recovery. At the end of the training year, you get to kick back a bit for a number of weeks.

Periodization Law #2: Go Slow-and-Long, and Hard-and-Short

In Periodization, the volume of training (weekly mileage) is always inversely related to the intensity of those workouts. After all, the harder you work, the less work you can do. So as your training progresses toward your competition phase and your intensity rises, your weekly volume of training miles must come down.

Periodization Law #3: Remember the 8-Week Rule

Central to Periodization science is that you shouldn't perform any type of workout for more than 8 weeks at a time. The human body reacts to the stress of training with an increase in natural anabolic hormones. These include testosterone (even in women), growth hormone, and insulin. These hormones help you adapt to the stress—in other words, become stronger.

But after about 8 weeks, fully adapted to this one type of stress, the hormone response to it fades because the body no longer sees that particular type of training as stressful. Continuing to perform the same type of training without the benefit of this hormonal backup will then create a state of overtraining. That's why, after 8 weeks, the training stimulus must be altered to create a different type of stress and trigger another hormonal upsurge. In this way, Periodization training has been called *natural doping* because it keeps your hormonal system peaked throughout the year. People get confused. They do low-intensity base training and think, "How can I get overtrained?" Well, after 8 weeks, even low-intensity exercise makes the body stale.

Periodization Law #4: Push Your Fitness Up Slowly

Instead of going out and doing a superhard workout in an attempt to get up to speed quickly, you have to take it slow with workouts that are in line with your current level of fitness and progress from there. Otherwise, you risk suffering plateaus, burnout, and injury. Workouts do not define your fitness; your current fitness dictates the appropriate level and intensity of your next workout.

Periodization Law #5: Don't Screw Up Phase 1—It's the Key

You can get very, very fit on Phase 1 alone, although it won't leave you at your tip-top peak. In fact, the biggest fitness gains are accomplished in this first and most critical phase. This is where the foundation of all fitness is created. But rushing Phase 1 and trying to attain a fitness peak too early creates an artificial ceiling on how fit you can get and may even set you back with burnout and injury.

Periodization Law #6: Train Slower to Go Faster by Burning More Fat

Although counterintuitive, starting your training with low-intensity aerobic exercise is the best way to run faster later. That's because it turns you into what I like to call a *better butter burner*—someone with a monster aerobic system loaded with muscle cells that have an enhanced ability to produce energy from fat. *Aerobic* means that you are going slow enough to give your body all the oxygen it needs, and an oxygen-rich environment uses a relatively slow-burning fuel such as fat more easily. When you increase your speed to where you can't meet your oxygen needs, your body reaches for a faster-burning fuel—carbohydrates. By training your body to burn fat, you solve three problems:

- You won't bonk, because your cells reach for less of the limited carbohydrate stored in your liver and muscle cells, leaving enough to last until the end of your race.

- You can eat less during your race—i.e., require fewer calories—because you can tap the unlimited supply of fat stored on your body. That will reduce the risk of gastrointestinal distress (cramping, bloating, gas, or worse).

- You produce less lactic acid, meaning you become less fatigued. Lactic acid is a by-product of carbohydrate combustion. An added benefit of your monster aerobic system is that when you produce lactic acid during a hard anaerobic effort, such as climbing a hill or speeding up to catch a competitor, that lactic acid will be used by your aerobically fit muscle cells as an energy source. So you feel stronger through the race.

Periodization Law # 7: You Must Simultaneously Build Metabolic Efficiency and Structural Fitness Integrity

In each phase of Periodization training, you address each of the Four Pillars of Health and Performance discussed in chapter 1, with close attention to building your metabolic and structural systems together. This ensures that your engine (your muscles, including the heart, and lungs) doesn't blow out your frame (bones and joints), which can greatly set back your training. For more details, see "Metabolic Efficiency and Structural Integrity: Why They Must Grow Together" on pages 58–59.

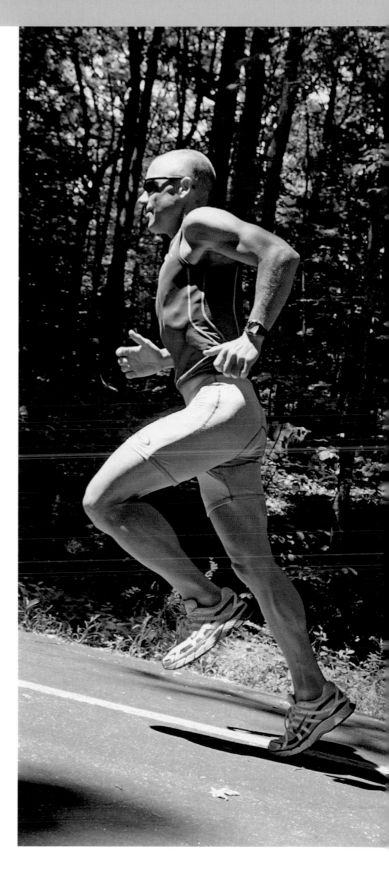

METABOLIC EFFICIENCY AND STRUCTURAL INTEGRITY: WHY THEY MUST GROW TOGETHER

Metabolic fitness refers to how efficiently your body turns food into energy for both exercise and daily activities. Metabolic fitness has made the terms *cardio* and *cardiovascular fitness* antiquated because we now know that the majority of the improvements in endurance that come from aerobic exercise occur in the muscle cells—not the heart (cardio), blood vessels (vascular), and lungs, in which improvements in performance occur relatively quickly and then stop. Within the muscles, however, the room for improved performance is more profound and takes longer to achieve. Yet this is where the vast benefits of training are realized.

The foundation of all fitness, whether your goal is to compete in the 100-meter dash or the marathon, is metabolic efficiency. Metabolic efficiency is defined as the ability to use more fat for energy at any intensity. It doesn't matter whether you're an Olympic athlete or a beginner age-grouper, the first order of business is developing your aerobic engine. This is the basis of Bob Kersee's gold-medal-winning success over eight Olympics; even his sprinters and jumpers first develop a huge aerobic foundation.

Base training upgrades the aerobic capacity of the cells by forcing (stimulating) your body to make three key adaptations, or improvements: increases in mitochondria, vascularization, and glycogen storage, detailed below.

METABOLIC ADAPTATION #1: MORE MITOCHONDRIA

Mitochondria are tiny energy production factories in the muscle cells where aerobic energy is created. If you like car analogies, think of mitochondria as the cylinders in the engine, where gasoline and oxygen are mixed and ignited by a spark, creating the energy that drives the moving parts. But instead of gasoline, mitochondria mix fats with oxygen to make energy.

The stimulus for growth of mitochondria is low-intensity exercise, done for longer and longer periods of time. The body will meet the demand for aerobic energy production by increasing the number of mitochondria in each muscle cell. This is how you turn your four-cylinder metabolism into an eight-cyclinder, supercharged monster truck!

Of course, a bigger engine needs more fuel to feed it. This brings us to the next key adaptation to low-intensity aerobic exercise.

METABOLIC ADAPTATION #2: VASCULARIZATION

Vascularization refers to your plumbing. As the demand for oxygen increases—in order to burn more fat—so does the need for the pipes that deliver it:

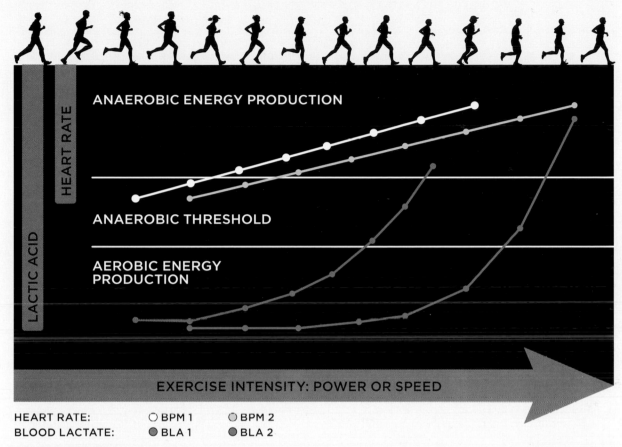

HEART RATE: ○ BPM 1   ○ BPM 2
BLOOD LACTATE: ● BLA 1   ● BLA 2

Illustration of improved metabolic efficiency using successive testing of blood lactic acid levels after 8 weeks of base training. The top two lines (BPM1 and BPM2) show the reduced heart rate as this athlete became more efficient after base training. The bottom two lines (BLA1 and BLA2) show lower lactic acid levels (a marker of carbohydrate metabolism) after 8 weeks of base training, indicating a greater, more efficient fat-burning metabolism.

capillaries, the smallest blood vessels. Again, the car analogy is useful. If the mitochondria are the cylinders of your aerobic engine, and oxygen and fat are its preferred fuel for best economy, then the capillaries are the gas lines and exhaust pipes. This "capillarization" of the muscle is the vascular infrastructure you'll need later when the increased demands of interval training take the working

muscles to their limits. They will require quicker delivery of oxygen and nutrients and removal of carbon dioxide and waste products, including lactic acid.

This process of vascular growth and increased mitochondrial density takes 8 to 12 weeks and requires that exercise intensity remains low. You can't see these changes, but they happen quickly if you stick with the program and resist the urge to surge. Intense exercise that takes you into an anaerobic training zone will interrupt your pursuit of aerobic efficiency. The improvements in anaerobic energy production are more limited; they will be addressed later, once you've achieved metabolic efficiency.

Developed hand-in-hand with the enhanced circulatory system and the bigger engine is another key upgrade:

METABOLIC ADAPTATION #3: INCREASING GLYCOGEN STORAGE

The limiting factor to all endurance efforts is that the carbohydrate stores (known as glycogen) in your muscles and liver last until the end of the day; otherwise you bonk (because your brain only runs on glucose, the simplest form of carbs). Your once-per-week long-slow distance (LSD) workout is designed not only to improve your ability to find and deliver fat to the working muscles to use as the primary energy source, but also to deplete your glycogen stores, so that your body (with the proper recovery nutrition), following the supercompensation principle, will be forced to store even more glycogen. Say, for instance, that at your current fitness level, your muscles and liver can store 1,500 calories of carbohydrate glycogen, and you nearly deplete it with LSD workouts; you will supercompensate and learn to store up 1,800 calories. Over successive weeks of LSD training, your body will adapt and increase its

storage capabilities to as much as 3,000 calories of glycogen.

So, while base training improves your ability to burn fat and spares precious glycogen stores, it also gives you a bigger glycogen fuel tank. This represents an exponential increase in your endurance potential—if you train right.

These adaptations are the bedrock of aerobic infrastructure on which you are going to build higher levels of anaerobic fitness later in the training cycle. In the end, your anaerobic fitness will be higher than it would be if you shortcut this base-training phase.

STRUCTURAL INTEGRITY

If you are going to build a more efficient engine, you also need a stronger, more efficient chassis to handle the increased power. This is where structural integrity comes in.

Structural integrity is how your body works on a mechanical level and refers to something that's often forgotten: your structural infrastructure, that is, the strength and flexibility training that creates resiliency of your muscles, tendons, ligaments, fascia, and bone. If they can't withstand the stress of your workouts, it will lead to a breakdown of your running mechanics and associated injuries that will limit your ability to train your metabolic system to its fullest extent.

Most runners, instead of having a deliberate plan to improve fitness, simply train their metabolic system until a structural breakdown occurs and an injury interrupts their training, creating an artificial ceiling to their metabolic fitness level. To reach your highest genetic potential as an endurance athlete, your joints have to work efficiently, and your connective tissues need to be hardened through the training process. By moving your mileage and strength programs forward slowly and following good recovery and flexibility routines, you will help this adaptation process occur. Think of strength and flexibility training as a shortcut to toughen the body against injury and improve running mechanics.

The fact is that metabolic fitness and structural integrity must develop together throughout the training cycle. As you ramp up the intensity of training, you will need a strong foundation of physiological and physical infrastructure. Too often an athlete in pursuit of optimal metabolic fitness is sabotaged by insufficient structural preparation, and when injury strikes and workouts need to be altered or suspended, their hard-earned fitness evaporates quickly. This is why you'll need a combination of gradual mileage buildup, weight training, stretching, and recovery, which as a group subject your body to supercompensation, in which it compensates for new exercise stresses with improvements in strength, power, and endurance. When broken down by exercise and then allowed to fully recover from it, the body will have a higher performance capacity than it did prior to the training period.

STRUCTURAL ADAPTATION #1: DAVIS'S LAW OF CONNECTIVE TISSUE ADAPTATION

The fact that connective tissue lengthens, strengthens, and becomes more flexible with use and shortens, weakens, and tightens with disuse is not new. In fact, Henry Gassett Davis, an American orthopedic surgeon known for his work in developing traction methods to extend and restructure bones, wrote about it in *Conservative Surgery*, his book published in 1867. "Nature never wastes her time and material," he wrote. "Ligaments, or any soft tissue, elongate by the addition of new material when under tension and, on the contrary, gradually shorten when they remain uninterruptedly in a loose or lax state."

The way that connective tissue incorporates the new "material" Davis wrote of is that every workout causes some breakdown of your connective tissue elements. Tendons, ligament, and fascia are all composed of collagen fibers. When they are damaged, the body lays down more collagen to shore up the areas of vulnerability. This functional scarring leads to a more resilient fabric of connective tissues able to withstand the high-stress activities later in the training cycle.

Stretching, use of the foam roller, and appropriate weight training are an important part of reorganizing these collagen fibers into functional patterns.

STRUCTURAL ADAPTATION #2: WOLFF'S LAW OF BONE ADAPTATION

More than a century ago, doctors such as German anatomist and surgeon Julius Wolff (1836–1902) noted that the principle of supercompensation applied to bones as well as connective tissue: "If loading on a particular bone increases, the bone will remodel itself over time to become stronger to resist that sort of loading," he wrote. Bone density increases when the body responds to stress by incorporating more calcium into your bones, making them stronger and more resilient to stress fractures. This process of bone hardening is accelerated and augmented with a gradual buildup of your mileage, adequate recovery strategies, and specific strength programs.

This is not only important to you as an athlete, but also for your long-term health. Men and women both need to be concerned about osteoporosis, the loss of bone mass as we age. Although two out of every four women will suffer an osteoporotic fracture in their lifetime (keep in mind that health experts expect 40 percent of the women alive today will live past 100 years old), one out of four men will, too.

You are never too young to put on more bone because bone mass peaks for the average person at age twenty-five—that is, unless you use resistance training to halt and reverse this trend as you age. Athletes are not immune, and in fact might be at greater risk because of all the calcium leached from the bones and lost in sweat. A study of well-trained competitive fifty-year-old male cyclists found they had the bone density of postmenopausal women. A weight-bearing activity such as running helps load the skeleton and make it thirsty to drink in more calcium, but it's not enough. I have met several veteran runners suffering from osteoporosis and osteopenia, its precursor. Resistance training, even in the water, pulls and tugs on your bones. These forces, along with a natural diet rich in calcium, will help mitigate the inevitable bone loss of aging.

STRUCTURAL ADAPTATION #3: PERFECTING RUNNING MECHANICS

The structural adaptations of Periodization training restore the flexibility and muscular strength lost in the sedentary modern world but needed for an efficient running gait. You need to strength train to develop the functional range of motion and power that let you move your body economically.

Bottom line: Engaging in strength training and habitual stretching before and after every workout not only helps you recover quicker, but results in a more functional rebuild of your connective tissue, stronger bones, and better mechanics than running alone accomplishes.

The Five Phases of Periodization in Detail

To recap, Periodization uses five periods, or phases, to prepare you for your goal. Each phase has a specific metabolic and structural conditioning purpose and can last anywhere from 4 to 8 weeks (but never more), depending on your objective and time frame, whether it be a 5k, 10k, or a marathon. In Periodization, every workout in a months-long agenda is performed with a specific objective in mind. I always tell my athletes, if you don't know the purpose of to-day's workout, take off your running shoes and go figure it out before you start your run.

Below, find each phase described in detail. Note: The training durations will be based on a 5-month training schedule for a marathon.

PHASE 1: BASE TRAINING

Duration: 2 months

Running plan: Long, slow, flat

Weight training: 2 to 3 days per week using light-weight exercises to isolate the small helper muscles around each joint that provide stabilization

Intensity: 55 to 75 percent of maximum heart rate (HR). (To measure your maximum HR, see the field test section in "Finding the Line between Aerobic and Anaerobic" on pages 68–69.)

Volume: Increasing

Daily nutrition: Speed up development of a fat-burning metabolism by matching your diet to the goals of this phase. By eliminating all processed sugars, including soda, candy, and baked goods, you can help your body learn to use its cleanest-burning fuel: fat. Consume healthy fats and lean protein to provide energy for the workouts and to rebuild your body afterward.

Metabolic focus: This 2-month base-training phase is broken up into two 4-week subphases—base 1 and base 2—in which training volume (duration and frequency) slowly increases in stair-step fashion. When you begin a new subphase, you're able to perform more work than the previous one. To visualize it, imagine the profile of two flights of stairs (see illustration on the next page). The first flight has three steps up and one step down to build in some recovery. The first step of the second flight starts at the same elevation as the third step of the first flight, in essence repeating the same effort but in a recovered state. The second and third steps of the second month are truly a buildup of your workload, as you are several steps higher than week 3 of base 1.

Key to success: Go slow. Gradually ramp up the miles with no more than a 10 percent increase per week. Be patient. Hold back. Fight the urge to pick up the pace, to increase intensity. Mark Allen, maybe the best runner in the history of triathlon, successfully demonstrated the benefit

ONCE A WEEK LONG-SLOW DISTANCE WORKOUT PROGRESSION

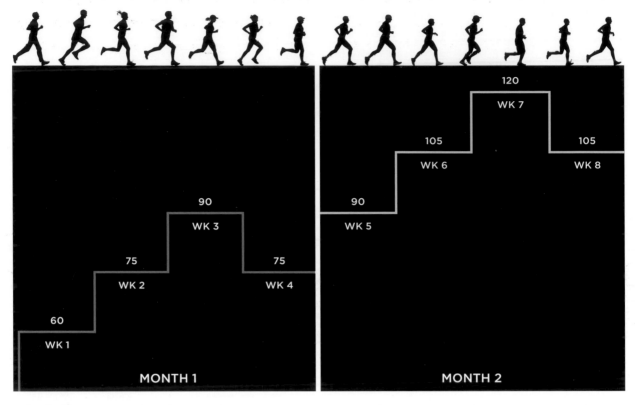

The numbers on top of each step represent the time in minutes of each long-slow distance (LSD) run performed once a week.

of this in the early '90s with Low Heart-Rate Training, a then-unique training method in which he deliberately kept his heart rate low, slowly building his base on his way to the last of his six Hawaii Ironman championships. Base training is all about low-intensity workouts at maximum volume—long-slow distance (LSD) runs.

Don't forget that the purpose of these gradual, stepwise increases in training time or mileage is to prepare your body and gain confidence for the harder work to follow. Physiologically,

you are building up the components of your aerobic foundation: stronger muscles, thicker tendons and bones, and multitudes of mitochondria with miles of capillaries, which are slower to respond to stimuli than your heart and lungs—all the more reason to throttle up slowly.

Face the scientific fact that you cannot do any high-intensity training while trying to develop your metabolic efficiency (base) in this phase. Intense exercise now will outrun your ability to process enough oxygen to burn fat, and you will go anaerobic (without oxygen): Your body, trying to keep going, then reaches for a quicker-burning fuel—your precious, limited stores of carbohydrates. Going harder will remove the stimulus for your body to develop more mitochondria and capillaries to build your aerobic engine. Later, you'll need to rely on them to stay longer in fat-burning mode at higher intensities of exercise.

Rest is also the key. Each 4-week subphase ends with a rest-and-recovery period, whether you think you need it or not. Science shows that you do. Three weeks harder, then one week easier. The fourth week is the all-important recovery week that calls for a significantly reduced workload (60 percent of the previous week's total mileage) that refreshes your mind and body, letting all your systems adapt to the stresses of training and come back even stronger. Warning: Don't train hard through your recovery week. You'll exhaust your body, stall your progress, and risk injury.

But recovery, as we've mentioned before, is not limited to this one week. A recovery workout should follow any hard or long workout, no matter the week or the phase.

Recovery doesn't necessarily mean sitting on the couch, although doing so one day of each week won't hurt. On recovery days, go out for shorter, lower-intensity runs, or cross-train: swim, do the elliptical machine, or ride the bike. Stay aerobically active, but lower the burners. A recovery workout doesn't produce additional stress; its low intensity is rejuvenating—like a massage. Recovery permits the body (and mind) to test the limits of athletic potential without falling over the edge into overtraining/underrecovery.

By the end of the 2-month base-training period, a prospective runner should have built his or her body up to the point where it can survive a 10- to 12-mile (16- to 19.2-km) run. For 10k runners, this would be 10 miles (16 km), for half-marathoners build up to 15 miles (24 km), and for marathoners, build up to 15 miles (24 km) on your way to your eventual maximum of 18 to 24 miles (28.8 to 38.4 km) in the next 2 months.

Whether you compete in 5ks, marathons, or Ironman triathlons, you are best served by developing a monster aerobic system. Building it requires extended periods of low-intensity exercise to force the above adaptations—and can be seriously sidetracked with even an occasional bout of higher-intensity work.

For finding your optimal fat-burning zone, see "Finding the Line between Aerobic and Anaerobic" on pages 68–69.

Nutritional optimization: In pursuit of metabolic efficiency, skip the sweet, sugary gels and hydration drinks during training and instead consume real food that contains healthy fats and protein (e.g., nut butters, nuts, jerky) and an electrolyte drink with little to no carbs. Limit processed

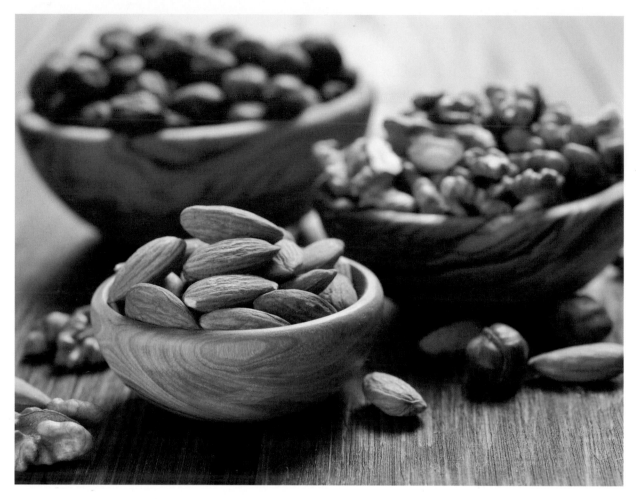

During base training, skip the gels and opt for healthy food. Nuts, for example, are an excellent snack food or training fuel.

carbohydrates such as whole-wheat bread in your daily diet as well and replace them with vegetables, beans, and legumes. This will speed your conversion into a better butter burner.

Structural focus: Weight training in these initial months is designed to isolate the smaller helper muscles that stabilize the pelvis, core, and shoulder girdle—that is, the skeletal anchors for the big prime movers that will eventually propel you forward. You'll train these smaller muscles with light weights (2 to 8 pounds [910 g to 3.6 kg]) in very specific movements to make them work better in their stabilizing roles (see the Runner's Dozen on page 150). This will create efficiency in your running gait by enabling you to maintain a rock-solid core when the larger muscles contract and pull and tug at your skeleton.

Light weights and higher repetitions stick to the overall low-intensity but higher-volume nature of this phase of base training. Accordingly, this is the time period when weight workouts are a bit longer but easy to perform. Weight training is best saved for your 2 or 3 shorter-run days of the week.

Stretching and rolling should become second nature and a part of every workout. They will help you adapt to the workouts and further enhance your ability to attain the efficient running mechanics you need to perform at your highest genetic potential.

Bottom line: Train right and develop your base with all the positive adaptations—structural and metabolic—derived from a scientific training methodology that will benefit you in all future athletic endeavors. In combination with technique drills, a sound flexibility program, and weight training (see chapters 2, 7, and 8, respectively), Periodization-based training guarantees you'll have a great foundation to build the highest levels of injury-free peak performance.

When you have finished these 2 months of base training, it's time to move on to a strength phase with low-heart-rate hill running and lifting heavier loads in the gym.

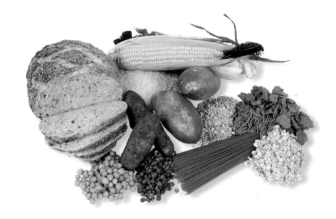

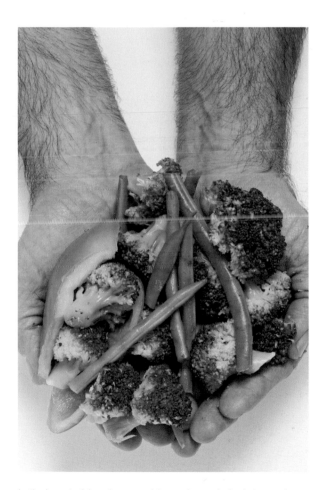

In the base training phase, avoid complex carbohydrates such as bread and grains, and instead include more legumes and vegetables in your diet.

FINDING THE LINE BETWEEN AEROBIC AND ANAEROBIC

The secret to vast improvements in performance in all areas of athletics is to start slowly, gradually developing the aerobic engine in a base-training phase. But how slow? Is there an aerobic sweet spot that maximizes the workout? How fast is too fast? Where's the line?

The line of intensity below which you are burning mostly fats is called the lactate threshold (LT). Say you are walking on the treadmill at 2.5 miles (4 km) per hour, going slow enough that your body is able to take in enough oxygen to combine with fat and make the energy necessary for that pace. As you slowly increase the speed on the treadmill and go faster and faster, there comes a point at which your body can no longer deliver enough oxygen to the cells to continue burning fat aerobically to remain at this pace. It's not that your lungs can't suck in enough oxygen; they adapt to training quickly. It's that your body does not have the delivery system (vascularization) to get it to the individual muscle cells, and the muscle cells themselves don't have the cellular machinery to use it and keep up that pace.

This is your LT. Up to this point, your body was burning mainly fat and very few carbs. The LT is the ceiling of your aerobic training zone. You want to stay below this line throughout the base-training phase to teach your body how to become a better butter burner. That is, burning fat at higher and higher intensities of exercise—and burning as few carbs as possible. There are two negatives to burning carbs: You have a limited supply of them and risk bonking, and burning them for fuel produces lactic acid. When the latter accumulates in the cells, it begins to shut down cellular energy production functions and you experience fatigue.

But linking your LT to a heart rate (so you can stay below it) is tricky without a clinical VO_2 max test, which has now become relatively affordable, although not often accessible. Instead, with a basic heart rate monitor, you can use the talk test or a field test.

The talk test simply involves keeping your running to a pace that allows you to carry on a conversation without being interrupted by labored breathing. Once you hit that point, record your heart rate and back off your pace a bit. That is your functional LT.

To perform a field test to determine LT requires you to have some moderate levels of fitness that would allow you to do an all-out running effort without getting hurt. Start with a warm-up at your long-slow distance pace and a 2 percent grade on the treadmill. After 10 minutes, increase the speed by 2 miles (3.2 km) per hour and raise the grade 1 percent every 2 minutes. Your heart rate should be rising steadily, and at one point between the increasing speed and elevation, you will feel like you can't go at that pace any longer. At that point hold on to the handrails, jump off to the sides of the moving belt, and quickly note your heart rate. This is thought to be about 90 percent of your maximum heart rate. Your LT is 65 percent of that heart rate. Your job in base training: Stay below that rate.

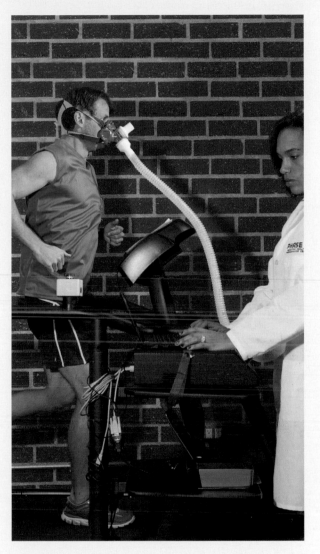

VO_2 testing, shown here, diagnoses a runner's current fitness levels and provides a prescription for training in the most productive heart rate training zones.

PHASE 2: STRENGTH DEVELOPMENT

Duration: 1 month

Running plan: Increasing intensity up to but not exceeding anaerobic threshold (AT). The AT is above lactate threshold (LT), where another shift in the energy production continuum occurs. Between LT and AT, your body is using an increasing percentage of carbs in its fat-carb fuel mix to meet energy demands. One day each week, do a low-heart-rate hill-climbing session to build strength.

Weight training: Target big prime-mover muscles using multijoint exercises with loads in the range of 75 to 85 percent of your one-rep max (see chapter 8).

Intensity: 75 to 80 percent of the maximum heart rate you achieve in a field test performed after you finish base training. (See pages 68–69 to find this heart rate zone.) You will use longer intervals up to anaerobic threshold.

Volume: Increasingly longer LSD runs

Daily nutrition: Stick to low-glycemic foods for your daily diet but add a hydration drink with a carb-protein mixture for longer runs.

Metabolic focus: After building your metabolic and structural foundation in Phase 1, your objective with Phase 2 is to raise your body's ability to tolerate the kind of hard work your goal requires—to, say, climb several miles without significantly slowing down. Your tools include low-heart-rate hill climbing, sustained long intervals ("cruise" intervals), and moderately higher-intensity training sessions than in the previous phase.

Technically, in Phase 2 you are trying to raise your AT, the point at which you begin to burn more carbohydrate than fat and produce lactic acid, a metabolic waste product. This is achieved with 15- to 20-minute cruise intervals up to your AT heart rate twice a week. The way to determine your AT is with the field test (see "Finding the Line between Aerobic and Anaerobic" on pages 68–69). The talk test will not help you determine AT.

Because what isn't trained gets detrained, long efforts are still part of the strength phase. Do a long-slow distance (LSD) run every second week in Phase 2. The mileage for this run should be close to your longest day of base training unless you are training for the marathon, in which case you will extend your biweekly LSD run to 18 to 20 miles (28.8 to 32 km), in 2-mile (3.2-km) increments. To prevent overtraining, in all cases follow the run with recovery time.

During this period, all runners will perform their peak weekly mileage because their intensity is about to climb, and so overall volume must start to decline per the basic tenet of Periodization: Weekly volume is inversely related to intensity.

Nutritional optimization: When attempting to increase lean body mass (i.e., muscle), eat adequate amounts of healthy protein with every meal. Your running and weight training will require that you eat approximately .9 grams of protein per day per pound of body weight. Continue to stay away from simple sugars and processed carbohydrates. Instead, eat lots of vegetables, beans, and legumes.

Structural focus: Strength-training workouts in this phase are shorter, with fewer overall sets and reps (i.e., volume). You will target the bigger muscles using heavier weights that still allow you to complete 10–12 reps using good form. Again, as intensity is increased, overall volume of your gym work must come down. As opposed to isolating the smaller helper muscles that function to stabilize the pelvis, core, and shoulder girdle, you will now target the prime movers themselves with compound movements. Your stretching and foam roller habits should be well developed by now and will play a big role in recovery and helping you avoid injury from these more taxing workouts.

PHASE 3: POWER CONVERSION

Duration: 4 weeks

Running plan: Cut mileage and add shorter intervals (6–8 minutes) that extend into the submaximal heart rate zones (above 85 percent of max heart rate, as determined by a new field test). If your goal race is hilly, add hill repeats.

Weight training: Shorter workouts using lighter weight loads (50 to 60 percent of your one-rep max) for quick movements to develop power.

Intensity: Intervals up to 75 to 85 percent of maximum heart ratefor 6–8 minutes with a recovery interval of 3–4 minutes in between

Volume: Reduced

Daily nutrition: Now you are a better butter burner who is able to burn fats at higher intensities, you will need to add more carbohydrates for the harder, more anaerobic workouts in this phase.

Metabolic focus: Training in this phase is all about putting your hard work to good use by converting your newfound strength into power, an essential ingredient of speed. Strength is defined as the ability of your muscles to contract and create a force. Power puts a time element into the equation; it's the ability to develop force quickly. Power training will now force your muscles to contract faster and apply the force to the ground in a shorter period of time. This faster ground-reaction time multiplies the forces that will propel you forward. Power is developed with shorter, higher-intensity intervals and short hill repeats. Intervals develop your anaerobic energy production systems by pushing the pace past the point where your aerobic system can take in enough oxygen to sustain the effort. Hence the word AN-aerobic—"without oxygen."

As your body begins to burn carbohydrates anaerobically, it produces lactic acid. Your body, primed by the on-again/off-again nature of the intervals, learns how to clear the lactic acid or use it as fuel for your struggling aerobic energy system.

Intervals will tax your metabolic and structural systems to the highest degree; therefore, it's essential to focus on recovery, which will help lessen the chances of getting sick or injured. Recovery starts with 8 hours of sleep per night. It also includes seriously practicing the recovery techniques you've already learned and honed. So you should stretch and roll religiously before and after every workout. And don't rush your warm-up or cooldown; they will limit the amount of cellular damage suffered in each workout and allow you to recover better afterward.

Nutritional optimization: Now that you have achieved metabolic efficiency and turned yourself into the proverbial better butter burner, you can safely add more healthy carbs (vegetables, beans, legumes, etc.) to feed the anaerobic energy system as you bump up the intensity.

Structural focus: Your weight training in this phase is all about getting the muscles to contract faster and move the weights quicker as you turn strength into power. You will use the same multijoint exercises as in the strength development phase but reduce the load to 60 percent of your new one-rep max for each exercise (see chapter 8) and increase the speed of your movements. This newly created power will help you pop over hills and provide the raw ingredient needed for speed. You can also develop power through the use of plyometric exercises.

PHASE 4: SPEED OR STRENGTH ENDURANCE

Note: Here's where the training program for 5k and 10K runners diverges from that for half- and full marathoners.

Duration: 4 weeks

Running plan:

- 5k and 10k: Volume (weekly mileage) decreases further as intensity is increased to develop speed.

- Half- and full marathon: Mileage decreases except for your long-slow distance run, which builds to 15 miles (24 km) for half-marathoners and 18 to 23 miles (28.8 to 36.8 km) before you begin to taper.

Intensity: High for 5k and 10k runners and moderate for half- and full-marathoners

Volume: Reduced

Weight training: Taper the weights to once per week using the same multijoint exercises as the power and strength phases but do higher reps (30) with extremely light loads.

Daily nutrition: Feed the body more carbs for hard days and lighten up for rest and recovery days to avoid weight gain as you reduce overall mileage.

Metabolic focus: Now you are ready to put the final ingredients in your fitness recipe for peak performance.

- 5k and 10k: Overall mileage comes down 1–3 minutes again, as does the length of your intervals, but intensity is at an all-season high with short intervals on the track.

- Half- and full marathon: For these distances speed translates into efficiency and fatigue-resistant muscles able to hold good form. This is accomplished with mile repeats on the track with the focus on holding form more than absolute leg speed. This phase is all about reinforcing good running mechanics in a fatigued state.

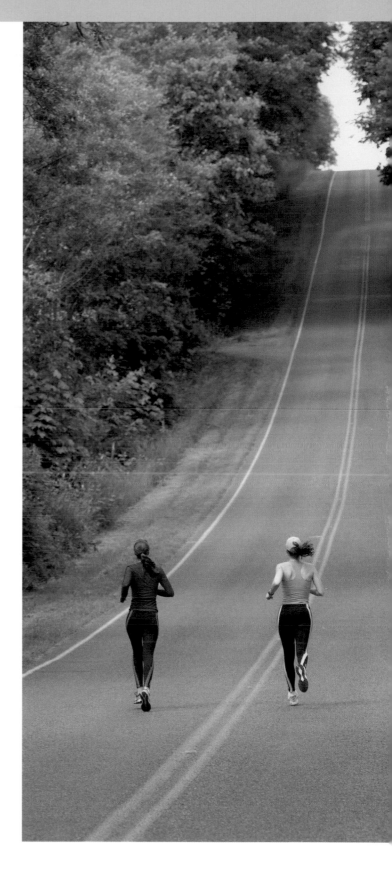

Nutritional optimization: Now that you have achieved metabolic efficiency and turned yourself into the proverbial "better butter burner," you can safely add more healthy carbs (e.g., vegetables, beans) to feed the anaerobic energy system as you bump up the intensity.

Structural focus: At this point in your training, approaching peak fitness with your running intensity at the highest point of your training cycle, you have to bring the weight-training intensity way down. The weight-room focus of this phase of training is designed to build fatigue resistance into your muscles. With high reps and low weights your muscle endurance will increase, but your muscles will not be tight and sore for your harder running workouts. Perform two sets of thirty reps with just 20 percent of your one-rep max weight. Build the reps by ten per set up to two sets of fifty reps by the third week of this phase.

PHASE 5: TAPER AND PEAK

Duration: 2 to 3 weeks, depending on your event's length and difficulty

Running plan: Reduced mileage, with hard workouts every 72 hours

Intensity: High

Volume: Reduced

Weight training: Light weight training continues once per week for the first and second week, with no weights during the week of the race.

Daily nutrition: Taper your calories, too, and limit them to all high-octane foods, including high-protein foods and nutritious soups with lots of vegetables.

The taper will make or break your entire training season. This is where all your hard work is actualized, but only if you understand the true purpose of tapering workouts. Tapering is not just allowing for total recovery; in fact, the week before your taper is a recovery week. Tapering is about using your newly acquired fitness to push your performance levels higher, but staying fresh. To reach the peak, you get all the systems firing together. This phase is like putting new wheels on your rebuilt race car and seeing how fast it goes and how well it corners for a few laps.

To make sure you peak, alternate hard, short efforts with lots of recovery, and keep the volume low. You work out just enough to sharpen up but gain a deep recovery that will leave you fresh. Beware of working out too much—you'll be fatigued on race day. It's a fine line that plenty of athletes have botched because they feel great, their legs have plenty of bounce in them, and they can't resist letting the horses run too much. You can walk the line successfully if you follow three rules:

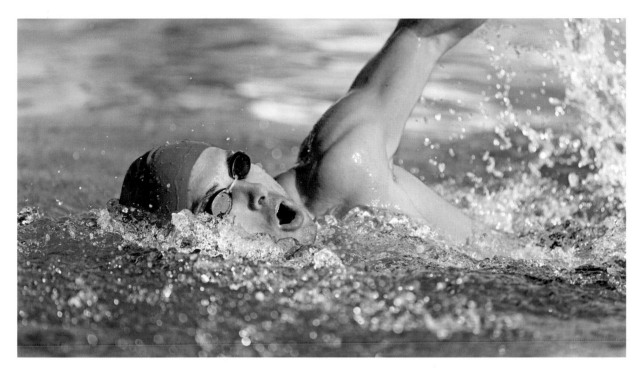

Swimming is an excellent cross-training activity.

- Rule #1: Avoid the urge to go for one last long run. You cannot develop any more fitness, but you can tire yourself out and sabotage the event for which you've been training for months. The stress levied on your body must now be unloaded for your top-level fitness to show up with you at the start line.

- Rule #2: The taper should be 3 weeks for half- and full marathons. For your most important "A-list" 5k or 10k, taper your workouts for 2 weeks.

- Rule #3: Maintain intensity, but cut training volume by 25 percent the first week, and then reduce it another 25 percent the second and third weeks. Shave duration from longer efforts. Reduce training frequency to every 72 hours as opposed to every 48 hours for the preceding training phases. You can hold a peak for a month, but not much longer, so when targeting several events, keep them close together on the calendar.

PHASE 6: TRANSITION

Duration: 2 to 6 weeks, depending on how taxing your last race or series of races was

Running plan: Unstructured routine of easy running and cross-training

Intensity: 55 to 75 percent of maximum heart rate

Volume: Low

Daily nutrition: Splurge a bit but make it with whole foods made with healthy ingredients.

After your event is over, spend the next 2 to 6 weeks in an unstructured active recovery period, giving the mind and body a break from regimented training. The length of the transition period depends on the length and difficulty of your training program. Swim or bike for fun, play tennis, or try a new sport. Give your legs a break but stay active so you don't lose all your fitness and gain weight.

The days of getting in great shape only to see it disappear because of burnout, long lay-offs, and injury are over. Year-round aerobic fitness and joint stability is the new normal, because Periodization lets you keep your mind and body fresh!

5 Nutritional Optimization

Real foods control your insulin, help you burn more fat as fuel, and help deliver optimal performance.

Training is only half the battle when it comes to achieving great results. Food is the other.

Just like with your training, a science-based approach to what you put in your body and when you do it has a great effect on your ability to achieve your athletic and health goals. My approach to health and fitness involves guided exercise and an easy-to-follow, "close-to-the-earth" diet. Both are designed for one singular goal: metabolic efficiency—to make you a better butter burner. We have discussed the importance of precision heart-rate training to develop your fat-burning metabolism in chapter 4; now it's time to dial in your diet to further serve this goal.

Food Is Fuel for Life— and Natural Food Is Best

All of us, especially athletes, need to alter our relationship with food. We need to view daily nutrition as the source of our life energy and focus on foods that further health, not disease. In recent decades, we've been told more about what *not* to eat than *what* to eat to stay healthy. Slowly, our relationship with food is changing as our food supply is being exposed as corrupted and unnatural. We are realizing that we need natural foods to help keep us healthy and make us stronger, leaner, and more resistant to disease.

Fact: Most foods In the grocery store have been processed to such a degree by the giant food corporations that they have little nutritional resemblance to their root food sources. Based on extensive and costly research from farming to processing to packaging, the food industries try to get us hooked with appearance and addictive combinations of salt, sugar, and fat. Natural nutritional integrity be damned! What's worse is that medical and health experts have unintentionally played into the "laboratory-food-is-better-than-nature" syndrome by incorrectly tarring eggs, butter, and other healthy foods as health killers.

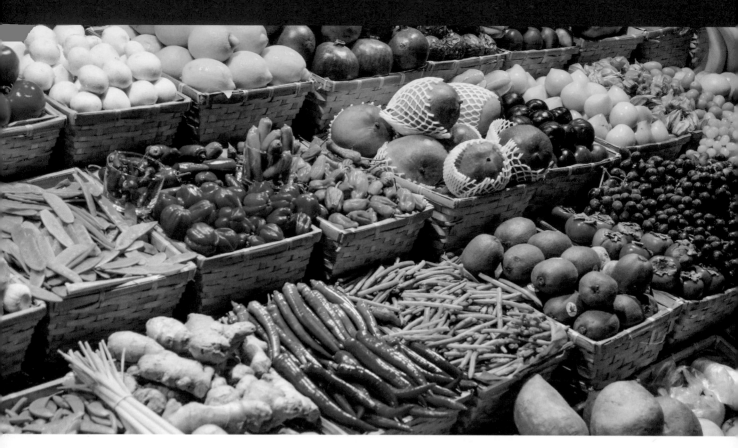

Healthy food is your fuel.

The key concept you need to remember about healthy nutrition is that you should eat foods that are close to the ground—meaning unadulterated and unprocessed. It's rare to find a food that comes out of the ground with unhealthy proportions of sugar, salt, and fat and that is damaging to our bodies.

Insulin Dynamics: Critical to Athletic Performance and Your Health

I feel the best diet plan is simple, science based, easy to achieve, and can be boiled down to one sentence: *Control insulin levels throughout the day and train your metabolism to be efficient at burning fat, not storing it.*

The problem is that we are constantly fighting the evolutionary forces that have programmed our bodies over millions of years to make and store fat to survive times when food scarcity was a constant threat. We have played right into our antiquated genetic predisposition by feeding ourselves an unnatural diet that encourages rampant production of insulin from the pancreas.

Insulin is released into your bloodstream to transport digested food into your muscle cells for energy production; the excess is stored as body fat. If you are not active and your muscles are not called upon to do any work, then all of the excess calories, whether in the form of protein, carbs, or fat, are transported to the liver and turned into fat.

There are only two ways to fight our body's built-in evolutionary tendencies: exercise and diet. You have read in chapter 4 that the first order of business for your workouts is to use low-intensity exercise, which reprograms your muscles to favor fats for energy production. Now it's time to focus on the importance of dietary manipulation during each of the Periodization phases to help achieve the athletic goals of each stage of your training.

KEEP THE CALORIES COMING TO STAY FIT AND STOP STORING FAT

Performance nutrition starts with sound daily nutrition. The value of good daily nutrition is analogous to good sleep habits; if you regularly get adequate sleep at night, but you miss some time in the sack because of a late night, you're still okay the next day. But do this too often and you will become chronically fatigued and rundown. Likewise, when you eat right every day and then miss a meal or snack here and there, your energy levels and your workouts won't suffer. To keep energy levels stable and ready, eat often. You must train every cell in your body to expect, receive, and use nutrients frequently (six times a day) throughout the day.

This cellular expectation is created when insulin levels drop a few hours after your last meal, at which time you need to feed your cells again with a snack. Your goal throughout the day is to keep nutrients coming at regular intervals so your metabolism keeps revving all day, burning more calories, and helping maintain a healthy body weight. At the same time, frequent meals keep energy levels constant to facilitate great workouts every time. But when you don't eat every 2 hours, your insulin levels wane and your metabolic motor goes into an idle. The result is poor energy levels, reduced calorie burn for the day, lackluster workouts, and potential weight gain.

PROVING THE FAT-BURNING PARADIGM

In the fall of 2013, a client of mine named Michael, a 40-year-old Los Angeles radio producer and a category 2 bike racer, decided to put me to the test. "Forster, you claim that I am now a better butter burner," he said. "For several months now, I've been dutifully following all your training and diet advice about the advantages of training my body to burn more fat as fuel. I have lost some weight and feel good. Well, this weekend, I'm going to ride in a 100-mile (160-km) bike ride with my wife and not eat or drink a single calorie all day—just to see if I can make it on water and my stores of body fat alone."

No problem. The next Tuesday, as expected, he came in happy as a clam. "Drinking water with only electrolytes, I escorted my wife all day long at a slower pace than usual—and felt great!" he said. "I even sprinted the last couple miles at the end!"

It's an extreme example, but the lesson applies across the board: This stuff works. You're safer, healthier, and perform better when you train your body to burn a higher percentage of fat to meet the demand for energy at all intensities of exercise and at rest (which we discussed at length in chapter 4). You last longer relying on fats for energy because every body—even skinny ones—contains an almost unlimited supply of energy in fat stores: 80,000 calories! (That blows away the skimpy 2,000 to 3,000 calories of stored carbohydrates.)

Eating and Training Your Way to Metabolic Efficiency

The untrained general public burns a fuel mix of roughly 65 percent carbs and 35 percent fat at rest (some metabolisms are even worse—burning as high as 90 percent carbs), and this is very inefficient. Your goal, instead, is to burn 90 percent fat at rest, and to keep burning fat at higher and higher intensities of exercise.

But training is not limited to physical training. Food training—what you eat—plays an equally important role in changing you into a

fat-burning machine. If you want to perform at your best and achieve optimal body weight and health, you must optimize your nutrition strategy—which means that you'll not only eat a good balance of natural carbs, protein, and fats, but you'll adjust the mix to match different training phases. Also, be aware that daily meals will be different from your post-workout recovery meals, and that those recovery meals must be eaten promptly after the workout to take advantage of a 15-minute "window" during which the muscles are more receptive to refueling. If you miss this window, you won't be fully recovered for the next hard workout. I'll discuss the window in detail at the end of this chapter.

To achieve metabolic efficiency and the better butter burner status, here's what you must do with your food intake:

BALANCED MEALS: MIX COMPLETE PROTEINS, NATURAL CARBS, AND HEALTHY FATS

Each meal will create a chemical reaction in your body that will either direct your cells to use food for energy or store it as fat. To create fuel, each meal must be a balance of fat, protein, and carbohydrates, all eaten together at once, not separately during the day. It turns out that the three work better together than alone, modulating the release of insulin and other chemical reactions that will either make you efficient or not.

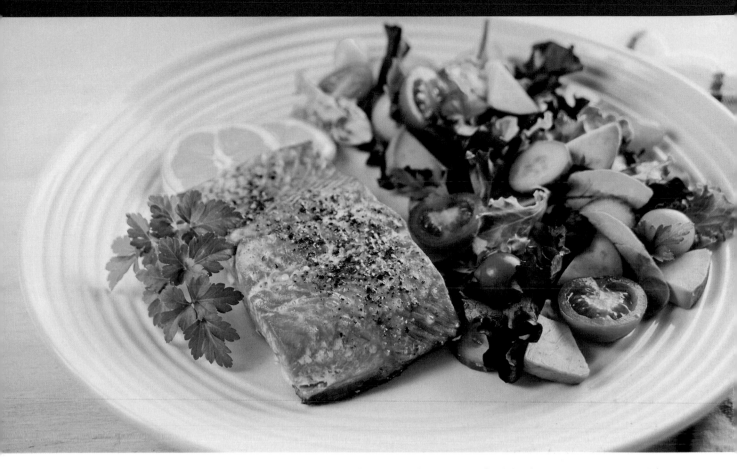

A balanced meal includes meat or fish (protein) with green vegetables (healthy carbs) and avocado (healthy fat).

The best foods are natural and whole, often characterized as *Mediterranean* in nature: lots of fish and low amounts of red meat, lots of vegetables, fruit, nuts, legumes, and minimally processed whole grains and other carbs and sugars. (See page 88 for more.) In general, these types of foods have a low glycemic index (GI), meaning that the body takes longer to break them down into blood glucose. In this way, low-GI foods help to balance blood sugar, lower insulin requirements, reduce body fat, decrease blood pressure, improve immune system function, promote longevity, and generally enhance well-being. Also, low-GI foods are the best choices for reducing inflammation, which is recognized today as the root cause of much of the body's problems.

Here's a breakdown of the three nutrition categories, including desirable foods and how much of them you should eat in each meal and each day. To help with your understanding of portion sizes, we will use a measuring device that you always have on you and is proportionate to your relative size: your hands. The proportions of each food category will vary within the different training phases.

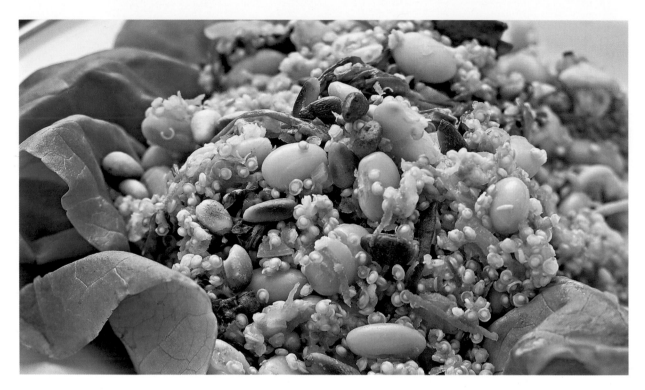

Quinoa and beans, pictured, provide good sources of plant protein.

Protein

- Complete animal proteins with all the essential amino acids, such as meat, chicken, fish, dairy products, eggs, plain yogurt, and whole-fat cheeses

- Vegetarian protein sources such as rice and beans, corn and rice, quinoa, soy, nuts and seeds, and nut butters. When you eat a diet with an abundance of veggies, they combine to supply all the essential amino acids necessary to make protein structures in the body.

How much to eat in each meal: 4 to 6 ounces (the size of the palm of your hand)

How much to eat each day: The general rule for runners is .9 grams of protein for every pound of body weight. This will vary from 30 to 50 percent of your total calories per day with Periodization of diet.

Good Fats

- Red meat and certain species of fish, such as salmon, tuna, mackerel, herring, trout, and sardines

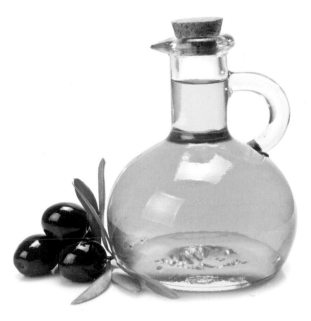

Olive oil and avocados are good sources of healthy fats.

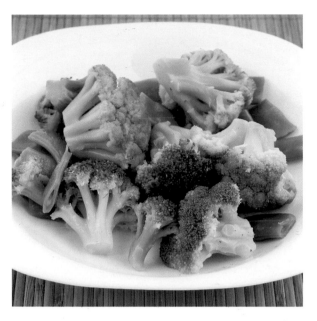

Eat two hands full of broccoli or another "good carb" with your meal.

- Oils such as olive, coconut, sesame, peanut, and safflower; avocado; nut butters and nuts and seeds such as sunflower seeds, flaxseed, almonds, macadamia nuts, walnuts, cashews, and pecans

How much to eat during each meal: Fatty meats and fish supply all essential fats needed for a meal. When eating leaner protein sources, add 2 tablespoons of the aforementioned oils to make it a well-balanced meal.

How much to eat each day: Athletes should consume 20 to 40 percent of their calories from healthy fat.

Carbohydrates

Your goal is to eliminate starchy and processed carbs, such as pasta, bread, sweets, and baked goods. Even if they are whole grain or whole wheat, they will delay or prevent your transformation into a better butter burner (because of blood sugar spike/insulin reaction and inflammation), especially in the base-training phase.

Good Carbohydrates
(Low-Glycemic-Index Carbs)

- Vegetables, including leafy greens such as lettuce, spinach, and celery

- Legumes, such as green beans, black beans, and garbanzo beans

- Nuts and seeds, such as quinoa, pumpkin seeds, and sunflower seeds

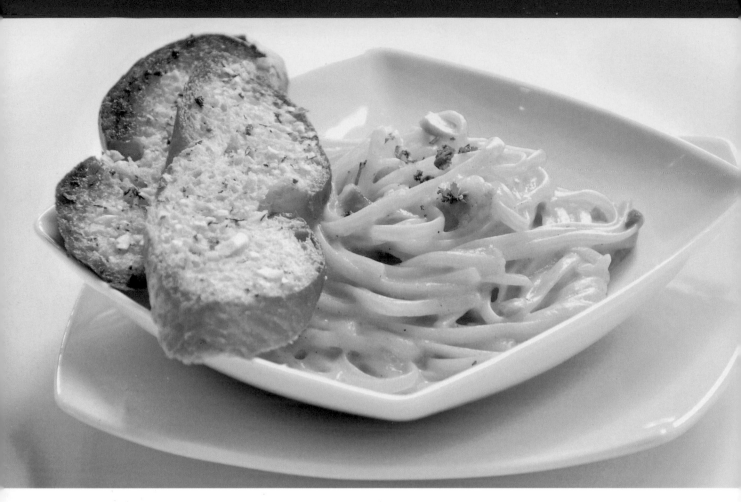

Pasta loading is out for runners.

How much to eat during each meal: Enough to fill two hands.

How much to eat each day: From 20 to 40 percent of your total calories should consist of low-glycemic fresh vegetables, nuts, and seeds.

Bad Carbohydrates
(High-Glycemic-Index Carbs)

- Find them in sugar, baked goods, candy, pasta, rice, crackers and potatoes.

How much of them to eat each day: If you cannot eliminate processed carbs and sugary foods, limit them to one handful and never eat them alone. Always pair high-glycemic carbs with a quality protein source to minimize the impact on your metabolism. The best time to eat refined grains and sugary foods, if you must, is after a balanced meal (meaning as dessert). Make them no more than 10 percent of total dietary calories.

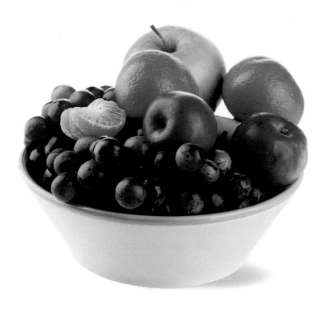

Despite the simple carbs, three servings of fruit earn a spot in your daily diet because of their vitamins and fiber content. Always eat after a meal to avoid the spike in insulin.

Note: Fruit gets special treatment. Although fruits are composed of mostly high-glycemic carbohydrate (fructose sugar), they also supply essential vitamins and fiber to your diet. So they get a special pass in your diet. Three servings of fruit per day is the maximum amount. Always eat fruit after meals, when the insulin response will be muted; or after workouts, when the fast-acting carbs are needed for recovery.

New Diet Rules for Runners: Beware of Carbo-Loading, Eat More Fat, Be Sure to Eat Breakfast, and Eat Frequently Throughout the Day

Our knowledge of food and diet is rapidly growing and changing. Some of the old rules that were long accepted as gospel have been turned on their head in recent years, such as "carbo-loading"—ingesting a great pile of carbo-hydrates the night before a big workout or an event to "pack" the muscles with glycogen fuel. It has long been a tradition in the endurance world. But it's wrong. Here's the correct eating strategy:

1. Avoid processed carbs. They prevent use of fats, spike insulin, and cause inflammation.

Processed carbohydrates include bread, pasta, rice, crackers, baked goods, and other sweets. (See "Wean Yourself Off Wheat: For Many Reasons, You're Better Off without Your Daily Bread" on pages 94–95 on the particular problems with wheat.) Processed carbs are dangerous for three reasons:

- Carbs stop fat use. Carbohydrates in your diet are counterproductive in your effort to improve fat utilization. If you put carbs in your tank, your body will reach for them as fuel before it reaches for fat to make energy for workouts and daily living.

- Carbs spike your insulin and put you to sleep. Example: If you eat a big bowl of pasta, the large insulin spike opens the cell windows and transports the carbs into the cells quickly, removing them from the bloodstream. That makes you sleepy or causes you to crave a sugar fix or caffeine to pick you up.

- Carbs create inflammation in the gut, keeping you chronically inflamed and bloated. Inflammation in the body produces excessive cholesterol. You will learn that saturated fat is not killing us; it's the carbohydrates that do that.

2. Don't eat carbs alone.

Dilute and delay the quick absorption of processed carbs and sugars by always eating them with a protein—such as peanut butter on rice crackers. Eat fruit only after meals containing protein. This mixture is one reason why the Mediterranean diet is so effective: It includes combinations of carbs and protein eaten together.

3. Don't fear fat—love it.

Recent research has exposed the big lie propagated by medical and nutritional science over the last 50 years: that dietary fat is making us fat, ruining our heart and blood vessels, and destroying our health. In fact, the opposite is true. Processed whole grains, the very food that we've been told is at the core of a healthy diet, is what is killing us.

Fat is far from the widow maker and heart-attack-waiting-to-happen that it's been made out to be for the past 40 years. It's an essential nutrient and a valuable fuel for athletes who have trained their bodies to burn it. This view is increasingly supported by research and many people in the know, the latest being an esteemed cardiologist writing in the October 22, 2013, edition of the *BMJ* (formerly the *British Medical Journal*).

Aseem Malhotra, MD, a British interventional cardiology specialist at Croydon University Hospital in London, wrote, "Let's bust the myth of saturated fat's role in heart disease." He says statistics suggest that decades of swearing off red meat, whole milk, and eggs has not only failed to reduce heart disease, but has "paradoxically increased our cardiovascular risks and that the real culprit are the sugars and processed carbs."

4. Don't skip breakfast.

Overnight, your metabolism goes down to idle, burning relatively few calories. When you wake up, you must jack up your metabolism with breakfast and start your engine burning calories right away. This will help you become leaner and perform better.

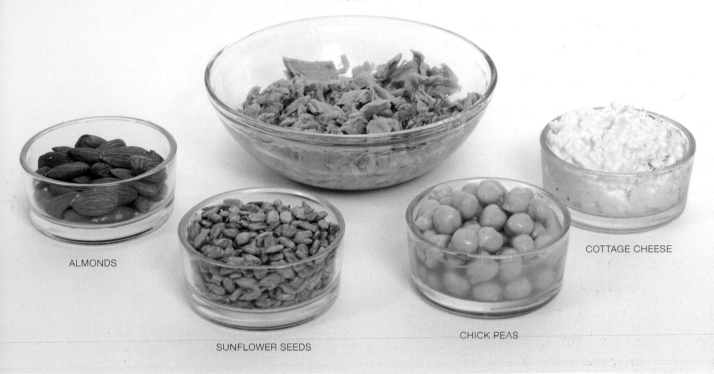

TUNA

ALMONDS

SUNFLOWER SEEDS

CHICK PEAS

COTTAGE CHEESE

Eat healthy snacks (100 to 200 calories) that are high in protein and fat but low in carbs.

5. Follow the 2-hour rule.

Eat every 2 hours. If you don't eat from breakfast until lunch, your insulin levels die down and so does your calorie burn. Between meals eat a balanced snack of 100 to 200 calories to keep insulin levels stable, which will prevent you from overeating at your next meal. Good choices include nuts, seeds, cottage cheese, tuna in oil, or yogurt. Never eat carbs alone for a snack. Break out the healthy snacks at 10 a.m., 2 p.m., and 2 hours after dinner.

6. Periodize your diet.

To maximize the effect of each training phase, you must alter the mix of nutrients to match your nutrition to the physiological demands of your workouts. Your daily meals and snacks and your post-workout recovery nutrition will vary as you progress through each phase of the Periodization schedule. This next section discusses this in detail.

Q: ULTIMATELY, WHAT'S THE BEST DIET? A: THE MEDITERRANEAN DIET

The diet plan that I recommend to everyone for healthy living—whether you are an athlete or not—is the Mediterranean diet, an eating pattern typical of Greece, Spain, and southern Italy that includes a balance of the following: olive oil, legumes, unrefined cereals, fruits, vegetables, moderate to high consumption of fish, moderate consumption of dairy products (mostly as cheese and yogurt), moderate wine consumption, and low consumption of meat and meat products. The great thing about the Mediterranean diet is that it's not only healthy but tasty, so it's very doable. Even better, after two decades of kudos and anecdotal evidence from longevity researchers, the Mediterranean diet's health benefits are now official. A first-of-its-kind study, published on April 4, 2013, in the *New England Journal of Medicine*, found that the Mediterranean diet reduced death rates from heart attacks by 30 percent.

The study, "Primary Prevention of Cardiovascular Disease with a Mediterranean Diet," included 7,447 Spaniards, aged 55 to 80, with heart-disease risk factors such as type 2 diabetes, obesity, smoking, and family history of heart disease. The researchers divided the massive test sample into three groups. One followed a regular diet and was asked to eat three servings a day of bread, pasta, potatoes, and rice.

The other two groups followed the Mediterranean diet, with one taking 4 tablespoons of extra-virgin olive oil a day and the other group consuming an ounce of walnuts, almonds, and hazelnuts per day. Both Mediterranean diet groups ate at least three servings a day of fruits and two servings of vegetables; fish at least three times a week; legumes, which include beans, peas, and lentils, at least three times a week; white meat instead of red; at least seven glasses of wine a week with meals (if they were accustomed to drinking); and were asked to avoid commercially made cookies, cakes, and pastries and limit consumption of dairy products and processed meats.

Sounds great, right? But, you may be wondering, how is this possible, given the large presence of carbohydrates such as pasta, bread, and cereal in the Italian version of the Mediterranean diet? It works because of the mix, the freshness of the food, and the portions. When mixed up and eaten as a meal, not in isolation, the low glycemic index of the "good" food (protein, fat, and veggies) slows the breakdown of the "bad" food—the high-glycemic bread, pasta, and cereals. Also, the market-fresh whole foods replace the calorie-packed processed meals and snacks Americans are hooked on. And then there is the portion of the carbs in the Mediterranean diet. They are not the supersized versions we've become accustomed to in

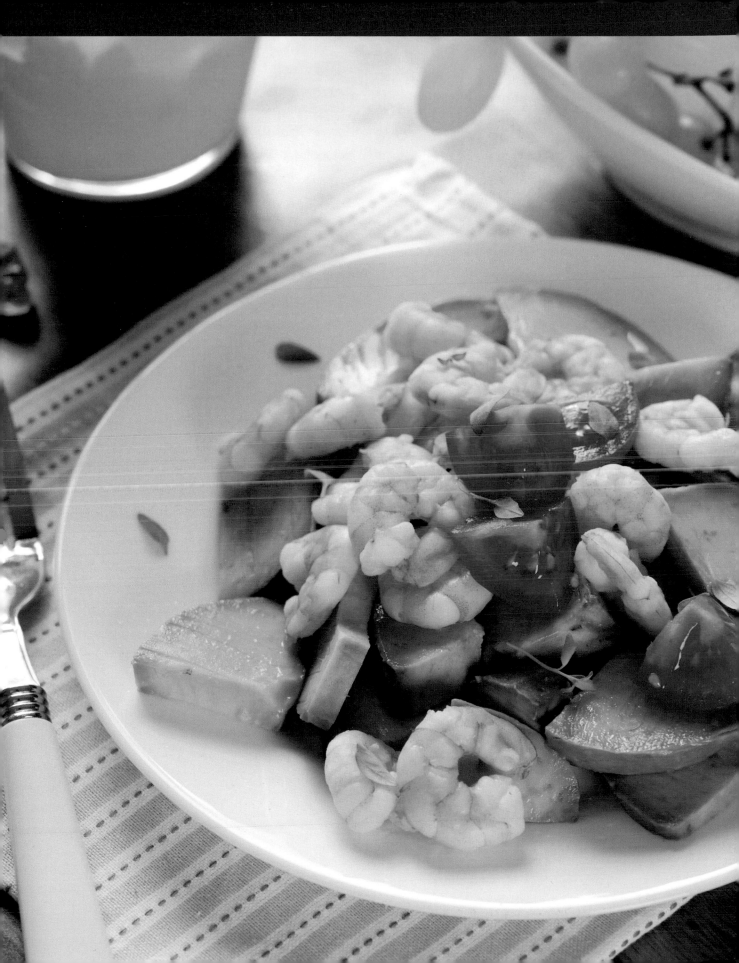

the United States; a few ounces of pasta in the Italian *primi piatti* (first plate) is easily dealt with by the body as opposed to the heaping bowl of pasta served in most American restaurants and homes.

Bottom line: The Mediterranean diet is quite healthy if you don't overdose on the processed carbs. Just make sure to load up on salad and protein when you dig into the pizza, pasta, and oil-dipped garlic bread.

HOW TO PERIODIZE YOUR EATING FOR OPTIMAL EFFECT

Because each training phase has specific goals and stresses your body in different ways in order to achieve desired adaptations, you must match each with an optimal nutritional intake.

Long-Slow Distance (LSD) Base-Training Phase

Approximate nutritional proportions:
20% carbs, 40% protein, 40% fat

The base-training phase is all about increasing your ability to burn fat to make energy. To help achieve this all-important goal, limit carbohydrate intake in your daily diet as well as before and during workouts. This will help train your muscles to burn more fat while you exercise. Instead of sweet gels, bars, and sports drinks, use plain water, nuts, nut butters, seeds, and electrolytes.

Also, limit your carbs during the recovery meal after your base-paced, shorter workouts. If you've stayed aerobic during your shorter workouts (90 minutes or less), you did not use up a lot of carbs, therefore, there is no need to replenish carbs. The exception is after your LSD workouts, which will have chipped away at the carbohydrate (i.e., glycogen) stored in your body. So after your LSD runs, you must break the low-carb diet of this phase to quickly restore glycogen stores before your next workout.

The best way to do this, ironically, is with carb sources that break down quickly into sugars—the very-high-glycemic foods you should typically stay away from. Examples include potatoes, rice, and non-wheat pastas, juices, applesauce, and so on. For those who continue to consume gluten in their diets, breads (even white bread) and pasta are good choices. If you have a sweet tooth, now is the time you can indulge yourself and consume candy but not chocolate, because the fat content will delay how fast it leaves your stomach.

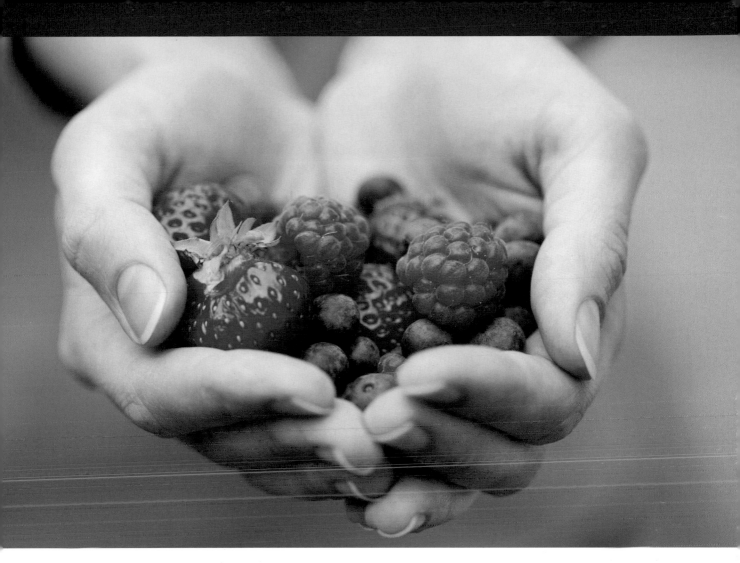

Limit an insulin spike by eating fruit at the end of your meal.

Strength Development Phase

Approximate nutritional proportions:

30% carbs, 50% protein, 20% fat

The major focus of this phase is to increase lean muscle. Accordingly, it is essential that you are taking in enough quality protein. Of the twelve amino acids, nine are essential to making healthy muscle tissue. Animal protein (fish, meat, poultry) gives you all nine. It's not as easy being a vegetarian athlete, because getting all nine amino acids from nonanimal protein sources requires you to become a serious amino-acid analyzer.

Power Conversion Phase

Approximate nutritional proportions:

40% carbs, 40% protein, 20% fat

During this phase, you are performing high-intensity activities, such as hill repeats and interval training, that burn carbohydrates, so . . .

- Up the carbs: Increase your daily intake to three handfuls each meal. Try to eat healthy, vegetable-based carbs, such as quinoa, garbanzo beans, nuts, and legumes. If you must have processed carbs such as bread and pasta, limit yourself to no more than one handful.

- Up the fruit: Increase fruit consumption to five servings a day. The vitamin C in fruit strengthens the immune system, which is heavily taxed during intervals. Because fruit is mostly sugar, it's best to eat it after the meal, so the other food groups previously consumed limit an insulin spike.

Speed or Strength Endurance Phase

- Approximate nutritional proportions for speed (e.g., 5ks to 10ks): 40% carbs, 40% protein, 20% fat

- Approximate nutritional proportions for strength-endurance (e.g., half- and full marathons): 30% carbs, 40% protein, 30% fat

With even-higher-intensity training in this phase, your carbohydrate needs remain at the highest of the training cycle. Remember that high-intensity workouts rely on carbohydrate metabolism. Continue the mix of nutrients of the power conversion phase.

Taper and Peak Phase

Approximate nutritional proportions: 30% carbs, 50% protein, 20% fat

This is not simply a period of recovery where your fitness evolves but also the time to put this newfound fitness to work. Although your overall workout volume decreases dramatically, short, hard workouts spaced out every 72 hours will help you find your race "gear." It is critical that you reduce overall calorie intake (10 to 20 percent) to match your calorie input to your reduced overall energy output; otherwise you will put on weight—not a good strategy for fast times on race day.

THE 15-MINUTE RECOVERY WINDOW

To ensure a speedy recovery and best adaptation from a workout, you need to take in both carbohydrates and protein—the former will begin to refill the stores of glycogen you've used up, the latter will jump-start muscle repair. Do this quickly. Science has established that there is a 15-minute window immediately following exercise in which the muscle cells are most receptive to absorbing these nutrients. If you let the window close without supplying them, all the hard work you just did and your recovery are compromised. So you should . . . *immediately gulp down something sweet.*

That will not only expand the cellular window but keep it open longer. Technically, pouring sugary, high-glycemic stuff such as fruit juices or recovery drinks into your bloodstream seconds after your workout is done will stimulate your pancreas to release insulin. So will the aforementioned sources that break down quickly into sugars: potatoes, rice, non-wheat pastas, applesauce, and breads. Make sure not to ingest much, if any fat, which will delay digestion. (That's why a chocolate bar isn't a good idea, because it contains too much fat. So feed your sweet tooth immediately but not with a Hershey or Snickers bar.)

Actually, to stimulate the best insulin response, researchers have found that the optimal recovery drink or food has a 4-to-1 carb-to-protein ratio. That little bit of protein kicks the pancreas into a slightly higher gear, putting out even higher levels of insulin, which now works to aid recovery.

From the time you ingested sugary stuff, you get another 30 or 40 minutes of open-window time. That gives you time to get in a quick shower and then eat a balanced recovery meal of protein, carbs, and fat in proportions dictated by the phase of your training. In about 4 hours, your glycogen will be fully restored.

Miss this window, and recovery slows way down. All this leads to the obvious question: What actually happens if you miss the window? It dramatically delays full recovery. Instead of carbohydrate being repacked in the muscle cells, it mainly floats around in your bloodstream. The liver then grabs a lot of it and turns it into fat for storage. It then can take as long as 24 hours to restore glycogen. The result is experienced as ravenous hunger the rest of the day and low energy the following workout.

WEAN YOURSELF OFF WHEAT: FOR MANY REASONS, YOU'RE BETTER OFF WITHOUT YOUR DAILY BREAD

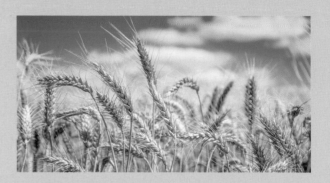

"Amber waves of grain" is lovingly etched onto the American consciousness. But what if all those millions of acres of wheat are actually hurting us?

Over the years, based on a growing body of research and anecdotal evidence, I've become convinced that wheat, a staple of our diet, is harmful. The body quickly turns wheat into sugar and spikes your insulin just as if you drank a can of soda. Furthermore, wheat creates inflammation, clogging your arteries and leading to everything from heart disease to cataracts. It is loaded with gluten, a protein many people can't digest well that has an addictive quality. It makes you obese, encouraging the development of a body-polluting "wheat belly," a term coined by William Davis, MD, in his 2011 book *Wheat Belly*. Davis says the big lump of visceral belly fat produces inflammatory signals that can lead to diabetes, hypertension, heart disease, dementia, rheumatoid arthritis, colon cancer, and foggy thinking.

The bottom line: Get rid of wheat and your weight drops and your health rises.

The problem is that wheat is not a natural food for us. People evolved over millions of years on meat, vegetables, fruit, and nuts and did not eat grains until 10,000 years ago. Our bodies simply were not designed to handle wheat's super-high glycemic-index level (it rockets blood sugar as

much as table sugar) and its high content of gluten. Let's examine both of those factors.

Wheat's almost-instant conversion to sugar leads to inflammation that then leads to clogged arteries and heart disease. That's because it encourages the growth of the most dangerous form of cholesterol—small LDL particles that can easily accumulate in the walls of the arteries, and your heart, neck, or brain, in a way that large LDL particles can't. Diet has a major influence on the volume of large or small LDL. Fat and protein have little to no effect on LDL, because they do not dump sugar into the bloodstream. Eating a three-egg omelet does not make you fat because it does not trigger an increase in glucose.

Gluten, found in many grains and seeds, namely wheat, rye, barley, spelt, kamut, and triticale, gives bread its pliability, elasticity, and spongy lightness and is used as a binding agent for baked goods. It's bad for two reasons. First, it isn't easily digestible for many. Roughly 30 percent of people of northern European descent are gluten intolerant, meaning that the body's white blood cells see it as a foreign agent, triggering inflammation. Chronic inflammation leads to a host of problems, from headaches, hay fever, and arthritis to sore muscles.

Second, it gets you addicted to eating. Gluten breaks down into substances called *polypeptides* that act a lot like opiate drugs, actually binding to the brain's morphine receptors, just like nicotine and crack cocaine. That makes wheat an appetite stimulant: It makes you want more food, healthy and otherwise. It is no surprise that obesity began accelerating in the mid-'80s, when "cut the fat and eat more healthy whole grains" became a national mantra and triggered an explosion of processed food products.

Because plant crossbreeding methods have increased gluten's density tenfold over the years and wheat flour is now found in everything from salad dressing to tomato soup (the average American now consumes about 150 pounds [680 g] of wheat flour each year), it seems like we're being programmed to become addicted to wheat—and to develop wheat bellies.

A decade ago at Phase IV, when I didn't know gluten from glutes, or that wheat could negatively impact your health, I started to notice a problem with our weight-loss clients, whether they were athletic or sedentary. Even after adjusting caloric intake and increasing exercise time spent in the optimum fat-burning heart rate zones, many clients remained pudgy and bloated. But when we reduced or eliminated wheat in their diets, the weight finally came off as expected. It turns out that many also reported fewer digestive problems, improved energy, fewer bodily aches and pains, and better mental focus, along with the weight loss.

Davis, the *Wheat Belly* author, reported similar findings. His patients who removed wheat from their diets lost weight, gained energy, slept deeper, experienced lower blood pressure and cholesterol levels, and even got some relief from arthritis and irritable bowel syndrome. Interestingly, he also opines that wheat ages you, encouraging the development of cataracts, wrinkles, and hunchbacks. That's because a by-product of its high blood sugar is advanced glycation end products (AGEs), the useless debris that stiffens arteries, clouds the lenses of the eyes (cataracts), and mucks up the neuronal connections of the brain (dementia). The older you are and the longer you've had high blood glucose levels, the more AGEs will accumulate and the faster you will age.

The more you hear about wheat, the worse it sounds. It's clear that the grain-fed pillars of old-school sports nutrition—the pasta, sweetened sports drinks, gels, and energy bars—must be replaced by smarter training and better workout food. Today we train athletes to use their own body fat to fuel their workouts and daily activities and direct them to low-glycemic, wheat-free foods that don't trigger inflammation or an exaggerated insulin release.

Breaking away from wheat will not be an easy task. Wheat products are everywhere—from the cereal and muffins you eat at breakfast to the sandwiches you have at lunch and the pasta you eat at dinner. In fact, even the labels on foods such as corn muffins, corn tortillas, and potato bread are disingenuous because they contain wheat and gluten. But knowing of the deleterious effects allows you to make an informed decision that can benefit your long-term health and athletic performance. Here are the healthy foods we recommend you eat during the Speed or Strength Endurance phase of Periodization training.

THE FORSTER EATING GUIDE

Here are some healthy food choices:

- Vegetables
- Raw nuts and seeds
- Healthy oils and fats, such as avocados, olives, and coconut
- Full-fat cheese
- Meats and eggs
- Non-sugary condiments, such as mustard, horseradish, salsa, etc.
- Flaxseed
- Spices
- Cacao

Limit your consumption of:

- Noncheese dairy, such as milk, cottage cheese, yogurt, butter
- Fruit, which is problematic because of the high content of simple sugars. The best fruit is berries because of their high antioxidant content.
- Whole corn
- Fruit juices
- All grains
- Soy products

Don't eat:

- Wheat products
- Unhealthy oils
- Gluten-free foods that contain cornstarch, rice starch, potato starch, or tapioca starch
- Dried fruit
- Fried foods
- Sugary snacks
- Sugary, fructose-rich sweeteners and artificial sweeteners
- Sugary condiments

6 Posture and Flexibility Assessment

Good range of motion and alignment are crucial to optimum performance.

In a way, this is the most important chapter in this book for injury prevention, and if I have learned anything about human nature over the years, it will be the least read. That's too bad, because almost every running injury that I see is the result of a body being out of whack, imbalanced, some muscle groups too strong or too weak, others too tight. It's usually just not because you're out of shape or lazy or suffering from an accident. It's because basic maintenance—stretching and strengthening—has been neglected. The good news is that it's easy to determine what the problem is—one look at a photograph of yourself can tell your story.

So that's what we're going to do here: Let you look at yourself to see where you are imbalanced, then have you test yourself with fourteen flexibility-assessment positions. Whether you're hurting right now or not, the assessments in this chapter—beginning with overall posture, then moving to part-by-part flexibility—will tell you why and what you must do to maintain a healthy, pain-free running career.

Posture Assessment

The definition of good overall posture is a standing position that allows you to use the least amount of muscular force to keep your body erect against the relentless forces of gravity. This requires your body's skeletal building blocks to be vertically aligned over one another.

You aren't born with body parts misaligned; that happens little by little over the years through work and play. Don't feel special—we all spend most of our lives in a forward-leaning, sitting position, typing at a computer or even riding a bike. Your muscles, such as the pecs and hip flexors, shorten and tighten to accommodate that position. Making matters worse, we exacerbate the kyphosis (excessive hump in the thoracic spine or the upper back) through imbalanced strength training at the gym. Too often runners work the front-of-body "mirror" muscles (pecs, biceps, abs, quads) with pushing exercises while neglecting the backside muscles (hamstrings, glutes, erector spinea [back],

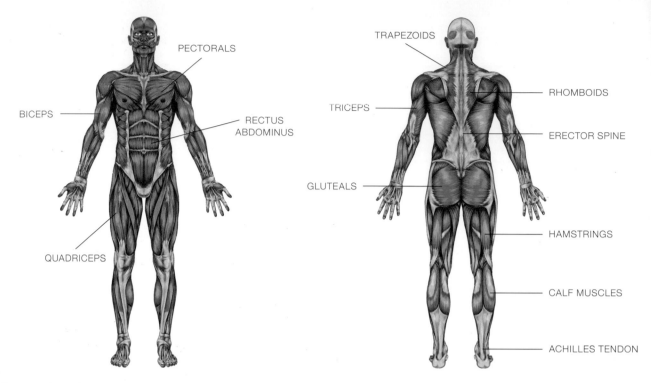

The muscular system

Labels on front view: PECTORALS, BICEPS, RECTUS ABDOMINUS, QUADRICEPS

Labels on back view: TRAPEZOIDS, TRICEPS, RHOMBOIDS, ERECTOR SPINE, GLUTEALS, HAMSTRINGS, CALF MUSCLES, ACHILLES TENDON

rhomboids), which are largely activated with pulling exercises.

Fully undoing the damage will take time, but when you start taking action, you'll quickly notice positive results. The remedy is actually pretty logical:

- Stretch the too-tight front-side muscles and strengthen the weak back-side muscles.

- And from this point forward, do twice as many pulling exercises as pushing exercises in the gym. Plus, give extra work to scapula stabilizers (shoulder blades), such as the rhomboids and trapezius.

LEG-LENGTH DISCREPANCIES CAUSE INJURIES

By the way, everyone I talk to is surprised when I tell them that a huge part of all overuse running injuries comes down to leg-length discrepancies—that is, one leg is longer than the other. There are two types: a structural discrepancy, in which a leg is truly longer than the other (in which case you may need shoe lifts), or the more common functional discrepancy caused by an asymmetry in your ilium, one of the two large bones that make up your pelvis. In other words, your pelvis is torqued one way or the other—and your goal is now to un-torque it.

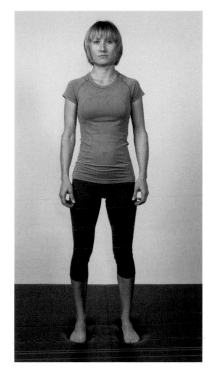

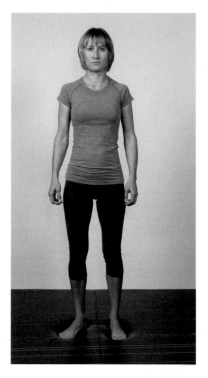

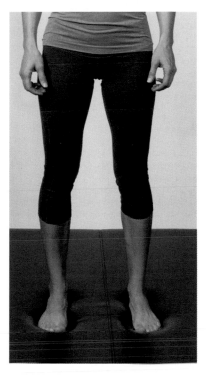

Do you see any asymmetries?

Right foot is externally rotated.

One foot is further from the midline (the line on the mat).

Because in my experience, the source of leg-length discrepancies are 99 percent functional and 1 percent structural, so nearly all of them may be fixable. I am convinced that the vast majority of overuse running injuries I treat are from leg-length discrepancies—especially if the injuries are asymmetric.

After all, ask yourself: If you have pain on one side and not the other when both legs did the same workout—why? If you look closely, you can see your own leg-length discrepancies in the mirror. Stand in the mirror naturally, not consciously correcting your posture. Now look at your legs and observe the following:

- Are both feet facing forward or is one more externally rotated—pointing outward? That could be the sign of a longer leg.

- Are both legs and feet equidistant from the midline, directly below your belly button?

- Is one arch collapsed (flat-footed) more than the other? It might be hard to tell, but which arch is closer to the ground?

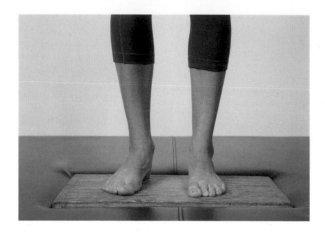

Right foot shows a collapsed arch.

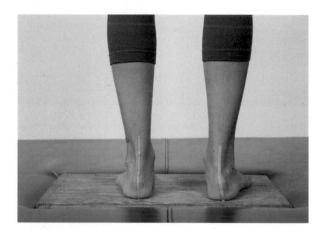

Right foot is pronated.

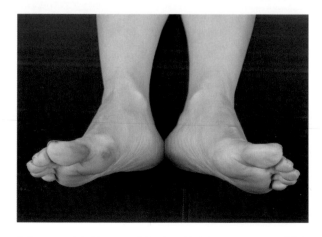

Calluses on right big toe and first knuckle joint.

- Inspect your toes: Is the knuckle of the big toe more enlarged on one foot than the other? And is the big toe on one foot angled outward more than the other? And is there a bigger callus on the inside ball of one foot than the other—or underneath the knuckles of the big toe on one foot? All these are signs that that may be the longer leg, whether the problem is functional or structural.

Even leg-length differences as small as ¼ to ⅜ inch (6 mm to 1 cm) will cause damaging forces to build up somewhere on the long or short leg, and can result in injury. If this is the case, go to an experienced physical therapist for a pelvic alignment assessment. He or she will work with you to create weight-bearing symmetry.

The bottom line: Even the worst postures are probably fixable if you are serious and vigilant. If you do all the stretching and strengthening outlined in this book (see chapters 7 and 8), your body will straighten up and your aches and pains will gradually disappear.

As I mentioned earlier, your posture issues are pretty easy to see. Just have someone take a picture of you directly from both the side and front (see below). Stand naturally without making any conscious adjustments.

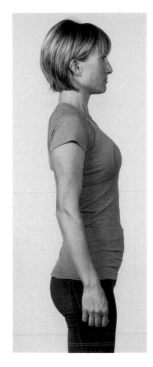

Good posture. Head held back with ear over shoulder, shoulders over pelvis, and arms at sides.

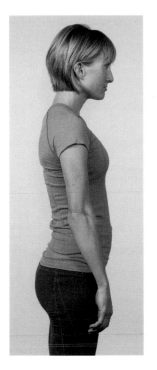

Bad posture. Head is thrust forward, shoulders slump forward, arms hang in front of body, and palms face backward.

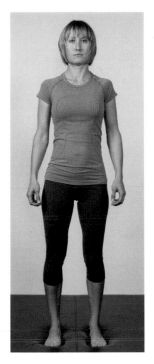

Good posture. Feet are pointed forward and are equidistant from the midline.

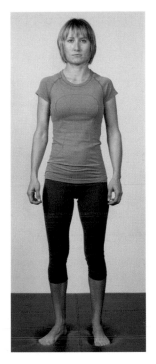

Bad posture. Foot on left points outward and farther from the midline indicating possible leg-length inequality.

1. Side View

Good posture: Your ears should be directly aligned over your shoulders, with the shoulders aligned over your pelvis, pelvis over knees, and knees over ankles.

Bad posture: Kyphotic spine featuring forward-positioned head; forward-slumped shoulders; swayed lower back; arms hanging in front of the legs with palms facing backward (instead of straight down at the sides with your palms facing your thighs); hyperextended knees that bend slightly backward.

2. Front View

Good posture: Head centered on level shoulders and level hips. (Shoulders can be slightly less than an inch [2.5 cm] out of line to account for natural right- or left-hand dominance). Knees are neutral—in-line with the ankles, not knock-kneed or bowlegged. Feet have equally well-developed arches.

Bad posture: Shoulders more than 1 inch (2.5 cm) higher on one side, asymmetric love handles (indicating one leg longer than the other), ankle bones collapsed inward due to overpronation on one or both feet.

Flexibility Assessment

To make the most of your body as a runner and to avoid injuries, all your joints must have a full range of motion. These fourteen flexibility assessment positions will tell you where to focus your attention most in terms of both stretching and strength (see chapters 7 and 8).

1. Forward Head Hang

What it does: Assesses the flexibility of your neck and upper-back muscles. The cervical extensors—the muscles that keep your head up against gravity—get weak and shorten after years of developing a forward neck posture, in which the head juts ahead of you. Causes include long hours of looking at a computer screen plus tight pecs, which pull the shoulders forward.

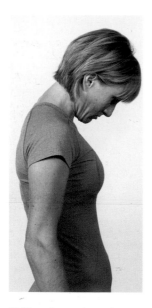 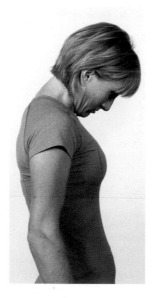

Tight neck muscles and incomplete range of motion

Better range of motion

How to assess: Drop your head down and try to touch your chin to your chest.

If you're healthy, you should be able to: Touch your chin to your chest with your mouth closed.

Implications for running: You'll have more stress and fatigue in your neck and upper back on long runs.

2. Chin Tuck

What it does: Like the forward head hang, it assesses the flexibility of the cervical extensors. (See image on page 133.)

How to assess: Suck your head backward like a chicken clucking.

If you're healthy, you should be able to: Suck your head back far enough to line your ears up with your shoulders.

Implications for running: You'll have more stress and fatigue in your neck and upper back on long runs.

3. Neck Rotation

What it does: Assesses the flexibility of the upper trapezius and sternocleidomastoids (the large group of muscles that wrap around the side of your neck to the clavicle).

How to assess: Turn your head to the side as far as it'll go without forcing it. The ideal, which most people probably won't be able to do at first, is to have your nose pointing directly sideways—that is, 90 degrees from the forward position and lined up over your shoulder.

If you're healthy, you should be able to: Turn your head to the side so that your nose lines up with your shoulder—not your eyes, your nose.

Implications for running: A limited range of rotation in the neck means the spine will be more susceptible to wear and tear over the years.

4. Shoulder Flexion

What it does: Assesses range of motion of your shoulders, which would be limited by tightness of your lats and the posterior muscles of the rotator cuff.

How to assess: Lift your arms straight up as far as they'll go.

If you're healthy, you should be able to: Touch biceps to ears.

Implications for running: Shoulder inflexibility does not allow you to hold good posture and maintain an efficient pendulum arm swing.

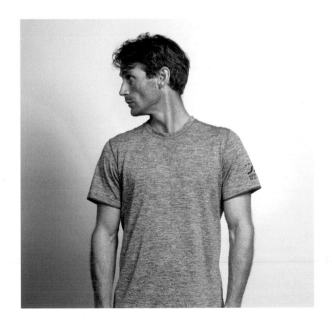

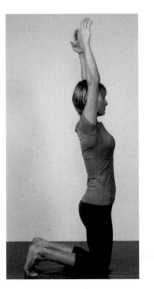 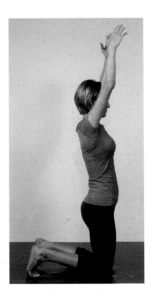

Full range of motion   *Incomplete range of motion*

5. Shoulder Abduction

What it does: Assesses the flexibility of your lats and shoulder joints.

How to assess: Hold your hands next to your hips with palms facing forward. Then raise your arms directly overhead in an arc (as in jumping jacks), with thumbs pointing upward as you go.

If you're healthy, you should be able to: Touch your biceps to your ears.

Implications for running: Not having the range of motion will limit the efficiency of your arm swing.

6. Standing Forward Bend

What it does: Assesses the flexibility of your glutes, hamstrings, and/or lower back.

How to assess: While standing, bend over and try to touch your toes with your fingers. If you can only touch your knees or mid-shin, one or all of these muscles is too tight (we'll sort these out in the tests that will follow).

If you're healthy, you should be able to: Touch the floor or toes (flat hands not necessary).

Implications for running: Tightness will limit your high knee rise and cause fatigue and tightness in your lower back on longer runs.

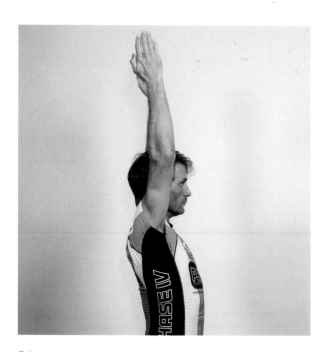

Full range of motion

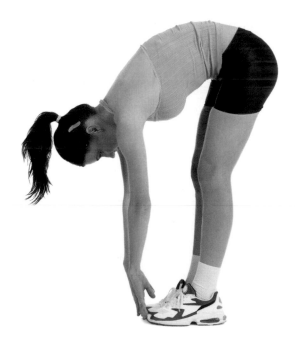

7. Double Knee-to-Chest Glute Stretch

What it does: Assesses the flexibility of your glutes.

How to assess: Lying on your back, pull both knees to your chest. If your entire butt and pelvis come off the ground, your glutes are too tight.

If you're healthy, you should be able to: Get your knees fairly close to your chest without your pelvis lifting off the floor or table.

Implications for running: Tight buttock muscles make it difficult to achieve the high knee position needed for good running mechanics. Also, your butt and hamstrings are the prime movers in running. If they are tight, they are weak, and so you lose power. Specifically, you'll have difficulty pulling your legs back under your center of gravity before they hit the ground, meaning you'll have a tendency to overstride.

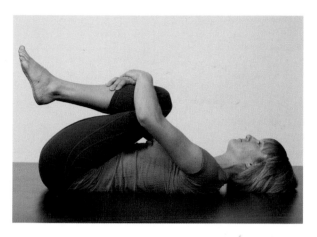

Good glute flexibility; butt stays on the mat as knees come to chest

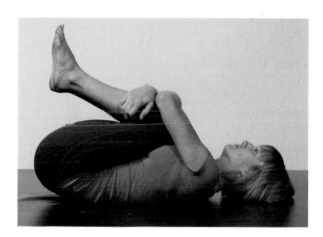

Tight glutes, butt comes off the mat

8. Thomas Test

What it does: Tests the flexibility of your hip flexors.

How to assess: Lying on a sturdy table on your back with your buttocks at the edge, bring both knees to your chest. Hold one knee to your chest while you lower the other leg down to the table. If the knee you dropped is hanging up in the air and not lying flat, horizontal with the table, or below the plane of the table, your hip flexors are tight. Now observe how bent your knee is on the lower leg. It should be relaxed, at close to a 90-degree angle. If it isn't, then the one quad that crosses the hip as well as the knee (i.e., the rectus femoris) is tight.

If you're healthy: Your thigh bone will lay perfectly aligned with your body and your knee will be bent at a 90-degree angle.

Implications for running: Tight hip flexors are weak, which impedes the high knee rise necessary for good running mechanics.

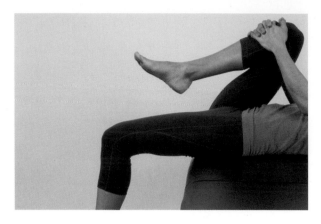

Good hip flexor range of motion; thigh lays on the plane of the table. Also shows good flexibility of the quad crossing the hip, the rectus femoris; knee is bent to near right angle.

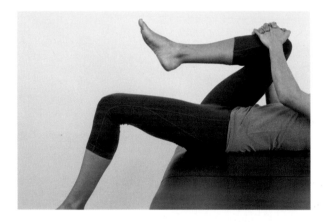

Tight hip flexors; thigh hangs higher than plane of the table

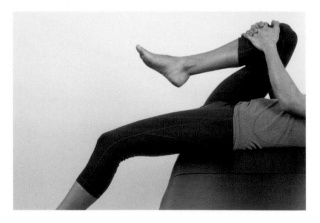

Poor flexibility of rectus femoris; knee cannot flex near 90-degree angle

9. Straight-Leg Raise

What it does: Assesses hamstring flexibility.

How to assess: Lying on your back, with one knee bent and the foot flat on the floor, raise a leg and loop a strap around the foot back by the heel. While your foot is relatively low, fully straighten your knee. Now raise the leg up while keeping the knee absolutely straight, and stop when you feel a definite stretch anywhere in the back of your leg—for example, the hamstring or calf.

If you're healthy, you should be able to: Bring the entire leg, with the knee perfectly straight and the toes relaxed and pointed toward the ceiling, to a 90-degree angle with your body. Anything less means your hamstrings are relatively tight, making you susceptible to knee, hamstring, and lower-back strain.

Implications for running: Tight hams mean you won't be able to achieve a high knee rise, which will degrade your rearward foot landing. You'll also lose power, because running power comes from the hamstrings.

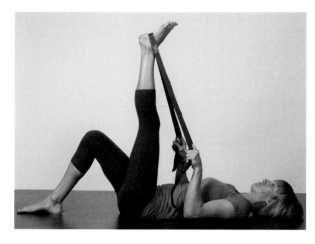

Good hamstring flexibility; leg raise to 90 degrees.

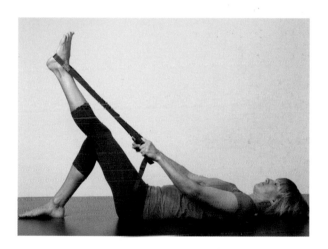

Poor hamstring flexibility; leg raise to 45 degrees

10. Patrick's Test

What it does: Assesses flexibility of the internal hip rotators deep in your buttocks.

How to assess: Lie flat on your back with your legs extended straight. Bend the left knee and place the left foot just above the right knee. Then relax. Then do the other side and compare the distance from the ground to your knee.

If you're healthy: Your knee should come within 12 inches (30.5 cm) off the floor. There should be symmetry from side to side, because asymmetry indicates that one hip joint is having more problems than the other.

Implications for running: Tight hip rotators make you susceptible to injuring the muscles deep in your buttocks, including piriformis syndrome and hip-joint deterioration.

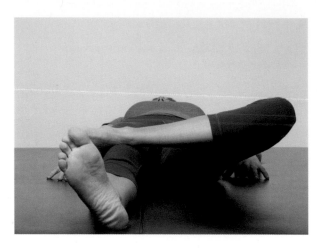

Negative test; shows good flexibility of hip rotators in left hip

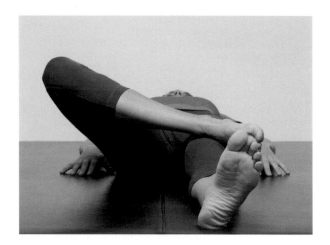

Positive test; shows tight hip rotators in right hip

11. Figure 4

What it does: Further assesses flexibility of the internal hip rotators.

How to assess: Lying flat on your back, bend both knees with feet flat on the floor. Place your right ankle on your left thigh just above your knee. Then reach down and push your right knee down while holding your left knee stable. Feel the stretch around your right hip.

If you're healthy, you should be able to: Look like the top photo. If you're tight, you'll look like the bottom photo.

Implications for running: Same as Patrick's test: Inflexibility makes you susceptible to piriformis syndrome and hip-joint degeneration.

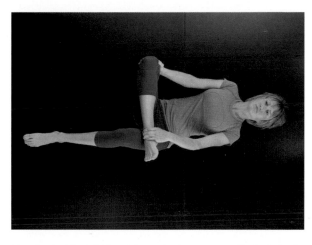

Negative test for left hip rotators; shin bone perpendicular to body

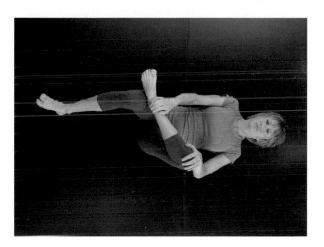

Positive test for tight hip rotators; shin bone not near perpendicular

12. Side-Lying Quad Test

What it does: Assesses quadriceps flexibility.

How to assess: Lying on your side with your hips stacked (perpendicular to the ground), bend your left knee and reach back with your left hand to grab the top of your foot close to your toes. Then pull your heel toward your buttocks.

If you're healthy, you should be able to: With your knee directly below your hip, pull your heel within 3 to 4 inches (7.5 to 10 cm) of your buttocks.

Implications for running: Tight quads make you susceptible to knee issues such as patella femoral pain syndrome and patella tendonitis. When the quads are tight, the patella won't track properly in the groove in the femur, scraping the sides of the groove and causing damage and pain.

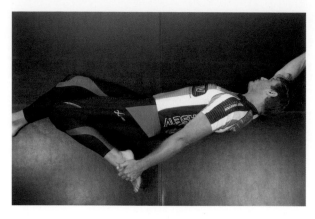

Negative test for tight quads: heel is within 3 to 4 inches (7.5 to 10 cm) of buttock and the knee is aligned directly below the hip.

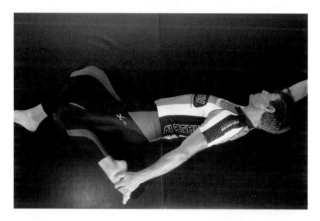

Positive test for tight quads: heel can't get within 3 to 4 inches (7.5 to 10 cm) of buttock.

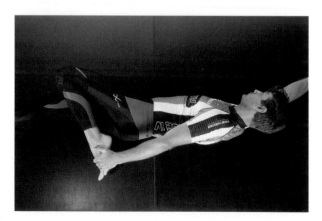

Positive test for tight quads: thigh can't get in line directly below the hip.

13. Long Sitting

What it does: Assesses flexibility of hamstrings, glutes, and lower back.

How to assess: Sit on the floor with your legs outstretched and try to touch your toes with your fingertips.

If you're healthy, you should be able to:
Reach for your toes. If you're healthy, you should at least be able to reach anywhere in the middle of your shin (not many people will be able to touch their feet). You should be able to see your pelvis angled forward (bottom photo) and an even curve from your lower back to your neck. (Any parts of the spine that are flat indicate tightness.)

Implications for running: A tight lower back makes you susceptible to knee, hip, and lower-back strain.

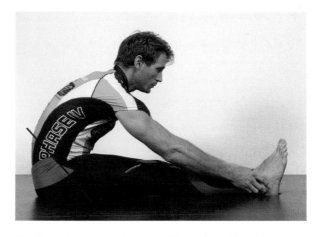

Positive for low back tightness; positive for hamstring tightness. Pelvis is angled backward and there is a flat low back curve, as indicated by the red line.

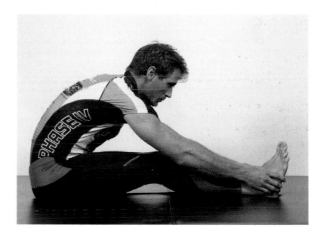

Negative for low back tightness. Pelvis is forward and there is a uniform spinal curve from tailbone to head.

14. Calf Range of Motion

What it does: Assesses the flexibility of your calves.

How to assess: Sitting on the floor with your legs straight and the bottom of your feet flat against a wall, pull your toes away from the wall.

If you're healthy, you should be able to: Pull your toes 2 inches (5 cm) away from the wall while keeping your heels against wall.

Implications for running: Tight calves can lead to overpronation, Achilles tendonitis, and recurrent calf injuries.

While you're evaluating yourself, note which tests were positive and which didn't work. Write the results down so you can emphasize those stretches later.

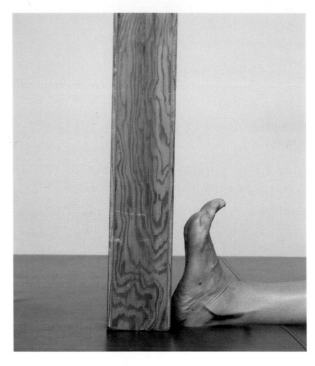

Negative test for calf flexibility

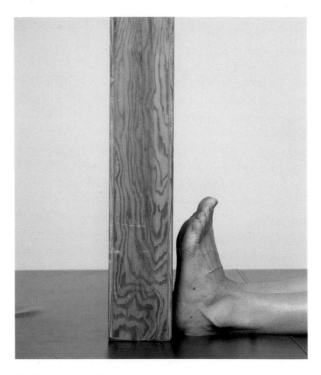

Positive test for calf tightness

7 Stretching and Flexibility

How 5 to 10 minutes a day of muscle and connective tissue lengthening perfects your form, and keeps the tightness, injuries, and doctors away.

When I first began working with Olympians in the 1980s, the number of gold medals won by individual athletes was directly proportional to the number of times a week I saw them in my clinic for what we called *health maintenance*—injury-preventive care that included stretching, massage, icing, and other recovery modalities. Jackie Joyner-Kersee came in the most and ended up with six Olympic medals. Florence Joyner, Flo-Jo, was a close second; she earned four Olympic medals.

The Olympians we work with today watched and learned from their idols. They often do much of their own body maintenance, working out tight muscles and scar tissue with foam rollers, softballs, and home ice baths. It's the rare elite athlete who doesn't do any stretching, which is often the most effective strategy of them all for recovery and injury prevention. I have worked with tens of thousands of athletes, from student athletes to pros and Olympic champions, and none have reached their highest genetic potential without a sound flexibility routine.

Unfortunately, even though it's simple, relaxing, only takes a few minutes, and can be done anytime and anywhere, average runners haven't gotten the message about stretching yet. Stretching is regarded as superfluous, ignored in the daily rush to the endorphin high. That's too bad, because inflexibility—i.e., a shortening of the muscles and connective tissue—is a drag on performance, an invitation to injury, and an aging accelerator. This is inevitable unless you do something about it—meaning you *must* stretch.

Regardless of whether you are athletic or not, you get tight as you age if you don't stretch. After all, even the most active people are inactive 22 or 23 hours a day, and inactivity has been shown to cause detrimental shrinkage at the cellular level throughout the body's structural tissues. Our mostly sedentary lifestyle leaves our bodies weak and tight, creating dysfunctional movement patterns that injure soft tissue and joints. The endless sitting in a slumped-forward position rounds your shoulders and trunk, shortening muscles in the front of your body and fixing your posture in a slumped position. In short, movement is life. Inch by inch, year by year, muscles and joints that aren't moved and stretched lose their range of motion. Before you know it, you start to walk a little more stiffly and bent over, becoming old before your time.

As noted, athletic people are not immune to inflexibility. In fact, running itself can hasten it, tightening the screws in your hamstrings, calves, and back and wrecking your form. Injuries rise as bones and ligaments get pulled out of alignment. Ever see runners and cyclists at their first yoga class? When doing toe touches, most can barely get their hands below their knees. They look like they're 80. That's because running, or any workout for that matter, creates damage to the connective tissue structures in and around the muscles. The scar tissue that results will naturally tighten if not stretched. Stretching helps the scar tissue mature into a functional scar, adding strength and preserving the length of your muscles and tendons.

For years, I've been obsessed with teaching athletes that the human body requires daily maintenance, just like flossing and brushing your teeth. I've given thousands of Saturday morning stretching seminars at my offices and with my partner bike shops and running stores. But to be honest, it is hard to get someone to follow through unless they are already hurt and desperate, or unless I grab their attention with the one surefire statement that every runner wants to hear: *Stretching will make you faster.*

Yes, you read that right: Stretching will make you faster.

Now I can't guarantee that stretching will shave 3 minutes off your 10K PR. But I can guarantee that you'll be injured less if you stretch, so you'll maintain your training without as much downtime. And I can guarantee that you'll recover quicker if you stretch, your posture and form will improve, you will run more efficiently, and you won't look like an 80-year-old when you walk anymore.

The bottom line, from a pure performance point of view, is this:

Flexibility is the first stage of good form, and good form translates to speed and fewer injuries.

For a good example of how inflexibility wrecks good form and slows you down, let's take body parts that you may not strongly associate with running: pectorals—specifically, tight pecs.

Tight pectoral muscles—most of us get them because we sit all day in a forward-leaning position and tend to favor front-of-body pushing activities over pulling exercises that work the back. This is a big problem for runners. Tight pecs wreak havoc with a vertical arm swing and pull your arm swing toward the center of your body, across your chest. This wrecks the critical vertical arm swing that turns your arms into a forward-motion pendulum. So tight pecs encourage too much side-to-side motion, which puts lateral shearing forces on your hips and knee joints, makes you run in a slightly more crooked line, and generally corrupts your ideal running form, slowing you down. The same story applies as you examine the flexibility of muscles and joints up and down your body.

Flexibility In-Depth

It might be helpful at this point to get a better understanding of flexibility. Technically, flexibility is defined as the range of motion of bones around a joint. Bones must have the freedom of movement to be positioned *just right* in the sequence of sport motion. This is what we call *proper technique*. When muscles have inadequate flexibility (i.e., they are tight), the opposing muscle will have to work overtime to put the bones in their ideal position. It's not hard to see why that can be a problem.

First, you may be so tight that your bones might move slightly out of coordination, in worst cases scraping on each other. That can lead to joint, muscle, and connective tissue injuries.

Second, it takes a lot more energy to get things done when you're tight. If you're inflexible during a race, you'll use up extra energy trying to maintain correct form, which will fatigue you earlier. For performance purposes, regular stretching gives you flexible muscles that allow you to run safely and push it harder with less effort.

Third, because you're doing less damage during your workout, you'll also recover quicker.

STRETCHING TARGETS CONNECTIVE TISSUE

Interestingly, stretching doesn't mean that you are stretching muscle fibers per se. You're actually stretching the *connective tissues*.

The red-blood-rich muscle fibers are elastic and will stretch without much resistance, but connective tissue doesn't. A thin casing of connective tissue surrounds each muscle fiber, wraps them into bundles, and gives them shape. White and glistening, these connective tissue casings are made of collagen, the same stuff that makes up tendons (which attach muscles to bones) and ligaments (which attach bones to bones at the joint).

While the skeletal bones provide the internal frame for the muscles to attach to and protection for the vital organs, it is the collagen connective tissue, or "soft skeleton," that holds everything together, giving the body its form and dictating how it functions. Where the muscle fibers dissipate toward the end of the muscle, the connective tissue gathers, forming a tendon, which attaches muscle to bone.

Bottom line: Connective tissue is everywhere in the body and vital to health, but most people give it little thought. Physical therapists spend their entire careers dealing with connective tissue and its dysfunction.

This gets us back to why we need to stretch the connective tissue. Like all structures in the body, connective tissue responds to the forces exerted on it. It thickens where it is exposed to stress and thins where it isn't. Also, it has a natural tendency to shorten over time where it is left unstretched. It is this connective-tissue shortening that limits the range of motion of the joint. A joint with limited range of motion operates with poor mechanics even in the available range of motion, which can lead to damage of the joint surfaces and other structures surrounding the joint.

So, to restore the natural length of the connective tissue, the normal range of motion, and therefore the proper posture and running form,

we stretch. The most effective way to restore length is slow, sustained stretching.

Here's an example of how poor flexibility can ruin good technique: In classic running form, the knee rise in the front of the body should be high enough so that the foot will strike the ground moving backward, gripping and pawing the ground like a bull getting ready to charge a matador. But if you have tight, inflexible butt and hamstring muscles, that knee won't rise so high, and your foot won't have enough air time to land correctly. This illustrates how an inability to touch your toes could result in a heel strike.

DIAPHRAGMATIC BREATHING

Central to optimum health and function is how we breathe. Proper breathing normalizes far-reaching functions including circulation, digestion, emotions, mental focus, and even pelvic floor function. Breathing is corrupted by injury, disease, anxiety, and smoking. Instead of deep breaths originating from the diaphragm muscle at the bottom of the chest cavity where the lungs are housed, muscles located higher in the chest and neck create shallow breathing. Instead, we need to breathe deeply using the diaphragm. Athletes and yoga students have learned to use deep breathing to control their focus and improve performance. If you can improve your breathing and harness the power of the breath, you will be a better runner and a healthier person.

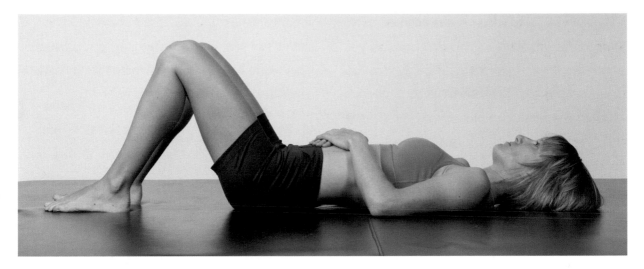

Practice diaphragmatic breathing, shown here, before working out.

Instructions:

- Lie on your back with your knees bent and feet flat on the floor at hip width apart.

- Place your hands on your upper abdomen and breathe deep into your tummy. Feel your hands rise and fall with each slow breath. Note any rise of your rib cage and work to minimize it so that all movement occurs in the abdomen.

Note: Before working out, use this breathing exercise to relax and allow the day's stress to leave your body.

Rules for Safe and Effective Stretching

To stretch is to de-stress, so savor it. A good stretch is long, slow, and relaxed. Stretching is not something you rush through. It's a time to relax, prepare your body, and focus on the workout to come. Practice diaphragmatic breathing and stretch before all workouts and at night. Here are the basics.

1. Stretch in a relaxed position.

Stretching is an act of relaxation, so don't force it. The muscle fibers must be relaxed for the stretch to effectively target the connective tissue elements in and around them. Accordingly, use stretching postures that promote relaxation and protect all the surrounding joints, especially those of the spine. Don't stretch leg and hip muscles under load—for example, in standing positions that force you to brace yourself, such as bending over and touching your toes or reaching back and grabbing your ankle. Instead, lie on the ground in positions that allow for muscle relaxation and easy breathing. For the upper body, the limb must be relaxed in a cradled or supported posture. Hit each of the major muscle groups while they are relaxed—not stressed.

2. Use the subsiding tension principle.

Muscles should be stretched slowly. Allow the stretch sensation to register in the brain and then modulate it by going deeper into the stretch or letting up based on that sensation. If the tension in the muscle increases while holding a position, then let up a bit. If the tension decreases, then move deeper into the stretch. Deep belly breathing, also known as *diaphragmatic breathing*, described on page 117, will further relax the muscle. Yoga focuses on deep breathing for good reason—it relaxes the entire body.

3. Use static stretching.

Dynamic movements mesh well with static stretching, but don't replace it. Although a few recent ill-designed studies found that static stretching reduced immediate power and strength output, decades of research shows that collagen lengthens best under long, sustained stretching and that a static stretch results in the most permanent elongation of the tissue. Stretching before workouts or competition allows athletes to execute the correct biomechanics of their sport. Indeed, my athletes set world records and won gold medals immediately following static stretching.

4. Stretch before all workouts and races.

The most misinformed view of stretching I've heard is that it is dangerous to stretch the body when it's cold. Shy of death, our bodies are never cold! Though collagen tissue stretches better when it's warmed up, it also stretches just fine at the normal resting body temperature.

To bear this out, just look at dancers; ballerinas don't go into the dance studio and run around to break a sweat before they stretch. They start the class at the stretch bar—and they aren't alone. Yogis, martial artists, and gymnasts, all with renowned levels of flexibility, first stretch, then warm up, and then stretch some more. As long as the stretching positions are safe and follow the subsiding tension principle, then stretching before workouts and competition is safe and effective to increase performance and help avoid injury.

Bottom line: There is no excuse for not stretching before a workout. In fact, we say that if you don't have time to stretch, you don't have time to work out!

5. Stretch after workouts.

Post-workout, the muscles are "pumped"—i.e., left in a shortened state with the blood vessels in and around the muscle laden with waste products such as lactic acid. Stretching returns the muscles to their normal resting length and promotes recovery by "wringing" the waste products out of the muscle as it pulls the connective tissue taut and staves off the dreaded DOMS (**d**elayed **o**nset **m**uscle **s**oreness). As a result, you recover quicker and begin working out again sooner and stronger. This prevents you from decreasing your flexibility as a result of training.

6. Stretch at night.

The quick 5- to 10-second stretches that you do before and after your workouts are designed to "release" your muscles to their normal resting length and maintain your flexibility. If you want or need to increase your flexibility, you must hold the stretches longer. Doing them later at night when your muscles and tendons are looser from the day's activity will create a more permanent elongation of the connective tissue and relax you for a better night's rest.

In summary, stretching is a crucial part of your workout plan. Done before and after you work out, and safe when done "cold," stretching prevents injury, loosens up problem tight areas before injuries occur, gives you the flexibility to run with proper biomechanics and technique, and serves as a mental and physical warm-up routine before exercise. Given that it feels good, is free, fixes your posture, and makes you look better in a business suit or running shoes, it's not smart to go without it.

The Stretches

The stretches below are not just for injured runners. They target all the crucial muscles to improve range of motion and performance as well as prevent injury. The 20 movements here are sequentially ordered in a specific routine, much like yoga, that progresses from lying on your back to lying on your side to all fours to kneeling and finally to standing. This gradually prepares your body for workouts and, afterward, for the post-workout recovery.

Do the stretches on both sides of your body to maintain symmetry. This can help you identify tight muscles on either side that require more attention. So, if you find a tighter side, work on it with a longer hold and additional reps compared to the other side.

When using stretches as a warm-up or cooldown, hold them for 5–10 seconds and do 2 repetitions of each. If the primary goal is to become more flexible, hold the stretches longer, from 10 to 30 seconds, and perform 3 reps of each.

1. Press-ups

An important exercise to increase and maintain lumbar extension and range of motion; press-ups are used to prevent and treat lumbar disc bulges. You may feel tight or sore in the low-back as you do this one, so only go to the point of discomfort and stop doing it if any pain radiates into your buttocks or lower extremities.

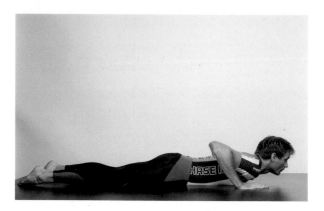

Instructions:

- Point your toes toward each other to keep your gluteal muscles relaxed during this exercise.

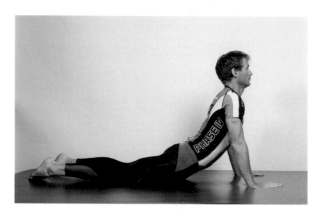

- Lie face-down with your palms flat on the mat near your shoulders, elbows pointed outward. Use only your arms to push your chest up. Extend as far as possible while keeping your pelvis on the mat.

- Don't hold at the top for more than 1 second before returning to the floor. Repeat up and down 10 times.

- Don't push past pain.

- Keep your head in a neutral position.

2. Pelvic tilt

Not a stretch, the pelvic tilt is a maneuver we do to be sure that your lower back is flat and safe on the ground before performing various exercises.

Instructions:

- Lie on your back with your knees bent and your feet flat on the mat hip width apart.

- Tighten your abdominal muscles and pinch your glutes together as you push your lower back flat into the mat. As you hold these muscles contracted, continue to breathe.

- Count to 5. Repeat 3 times.

3. Pelvic rotation

This stretch, plus the pretzel that follows, addresses the buttock muscles and is critical to avoiding injury. More than 50 percent of the running injuries we see are related to buttock and hip dysfunction.

Instructions:

- Lie on your back with your knees bent and your feet flat on the mat hip width apart, arms extended and even with shoulders.

- Cross your right leg over your left, knee over knee.

- Drop both legs to the right side, and slide them up toward your head as they maintain contact with the ground.

- Keep both shoulders on the mat and turn your head to the opposite direction. Breathe and hold for a count of 5. As you return your legs back to the start position, resume a pelvic tilt. Perform 2 repetitions on each side.

Note: Keep the foot of the bottom leg in contact with the mat throughout the stretch, and don't scoot your hips to the side before dropping your knees over.

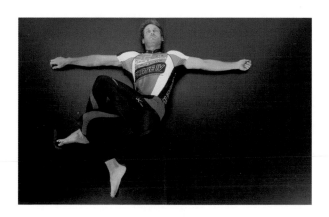

4. Pretzel

The pretzel specifically addresses tightness in the deep rotators of the hip, an area where common running injuries originate. It is the most preventive stretch for piriformis syndrome, a neuromuscular disorder that causes pain down the sciatic nerve in your leg when the piriformis muscle compresses it.

Instructions:

- Lie on your back with your knees bent and your feet flat on the mat hip width apart.

- Do a pelvic tilt and cross your right leg over your left, knee over knee.

- Place your right and left hands on your right knee.

- Pull your right knee toward your left shoulder. Breathe and hold for 5 seconds.

- Repeat with your left leg over your right leg. Do 2 reps on each side.

Note: Keep your shoulders pulled back during this stretch. As long as you are pulling your top knee toward the opposite shoulder, it's okay to rotate the leg by pulling more on the knee.

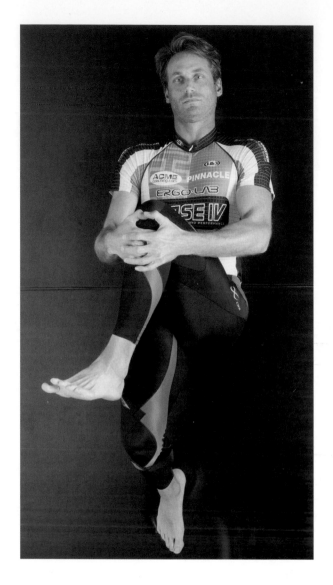

5. Figure 4

This is an important stretch to maintain hip range of motion and prevent hip joint deterioration. It's also important because it stretches the rotator muscles deep in the buttocks. Note: If you have an unequal range of motion in one hip or the other, spend extra time stretching the tight hip.

Instructions:

- Lie on your back with your knees bent and your feet flat on the mat hip width apart.

- Do a pelvic tilt and place your right ankle on your left knee.

- Use your right hand to push your right knee away. Breathe and hold for 5 seconds.

- Switch legs and repeat. Keep your pelvis symmetrical throughout the stretch. Do 2 reps on each side.

Note: To increase the stretch, lift your left leg off the floor and hold it behind the knee as you push down with your right hand. Also try the stretch as above, but instead of pushing the right knee away, pull both legs toward your trunk to increase the stretch.

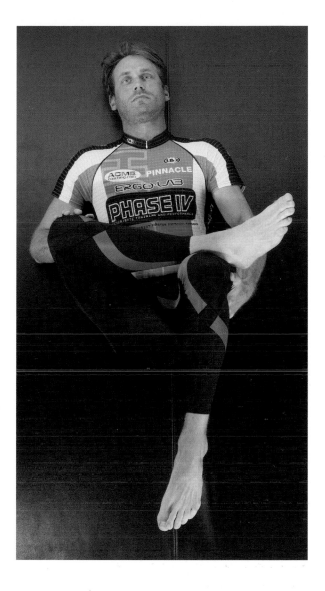

6. Supine Adductor

Place your hands on the insides of your knees and apply light pressure, feeling the stretch at the inner thigh as your legs remain airborne.

Instructions:

- Lie on your back and perform a pelvic tilt, raising your thighs so they are perpendicular to your body at 90 degrees. Bend your knees, feet up in the air.

- Place your hands on the inside of your knees and let both knees and feet drop outward. Apply light pressure with your hands. You should feel the stretch at your inner thigh. Hold for a count of 10. Repeat twice.

Note: Keep your knees and hips bent at right angles.

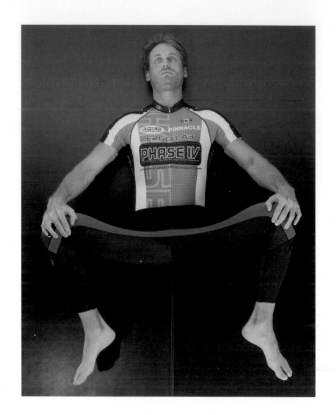

7. Side-Lying Quad Stretch

Doing this stretch regularly is the single most important thing you can do to avoid knee injuries as you continue running. The quadriceps tighten over time and create excessive wear on the kneecap as it tracks between the condyles (the two round prominences at the bottom of the thigh bone) of the femur. If left unstretched, runners are susceptible to patella tendonitis, or "runner's knee," and early arthritic changes in the knee. This is the one stretch that we will allow runners to work with, not through, some discomfort, because the stretch serves the greater good of improving the joint mechanics. This means that you need to continue doing this stretch when the discomfort is merely mild, doesn't worsen with each repetition, and you don't experience more pain in daily activities such as climbing stairs or squatting after doing this stretch.

Instructions:

- Lie on your side with your head on your arm and your hips perpendicular to the floor.

- Bend your top knee and grab your shoelaces and toes behind you with the same-side hand. Pull your heel to your buttocks. Feel the stretch at the front of your thighs. Hold for a count of 10. Do 2 reps on each side.

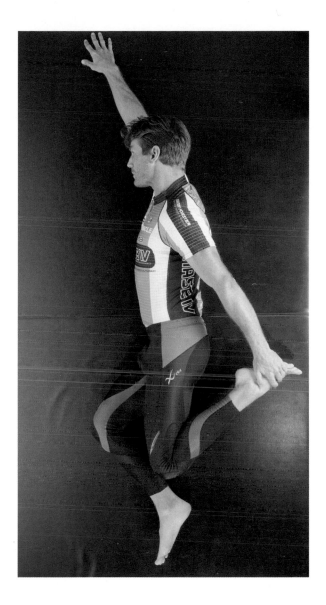

Note: During the stretch, keep your abdominals firm to support your back. Also, keep your top leg level with your heel behind you and don't hyperextend your back. Keep your shoulders and hips stacked. You should not be able to see your stretched knee if you look down your body.

8. Catback

This is an important exercise to stretch the muscles around your spine from your neck all the way down to your sacrum (the fused vertebrae at the bottom of the spine). If at any time you feel unbalanced, move your knees farther apart.

Instructions:

- Start on your hands and knees, with your hands below your shoulders and your knees below your hips.

- Arch up the middle of your back into a mild stretch and relax your head and neck. Feel the stretch in your mid-back. Make sure your arms and thighs are vertical. Hold for a count of 10.

- Return to the original position, and repeat.

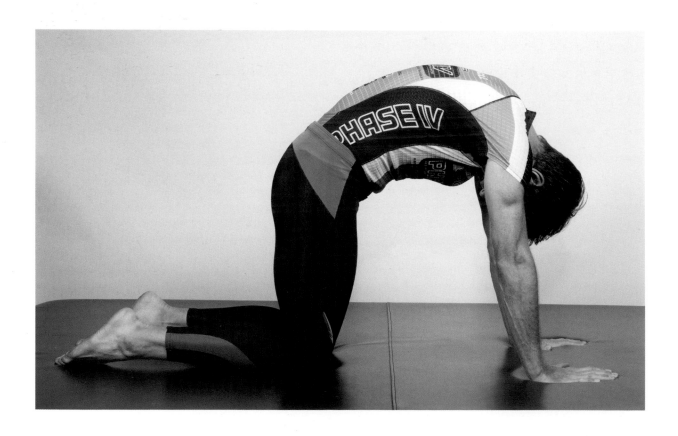

9. Prayer Position

This movement stretches the hard-to-get-to muscles in your lower back that are susceptible to tightening in runners (especially those with a leg-length discrepancy).

Instructions:

- From the catback position, simply rock yourself back toward your calf muscles, bend your elbows, and aim your chin in-between your knees.

- Walk both hands over to the left above your head, anchor your right hand to the mat with your left hand, and pull back through your left buttock. Feel the stretch anywhere from your right lat into your lower back. Over time, as you stretch out your lat, the stretch will focus on the lower-back muscle.

- Hold for a count of 10 and repeat on the other side.

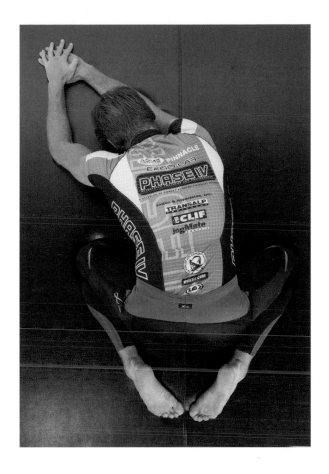

10. Kneeling Hip Flexor Stretch

The hip flexors will shorten with time with continued running, often causing lower-back pain and injury. Keeping them stretched out prevents groin injuries and spinal problems.

Instructions:

- Kneel on your right knee with your left foot at arm's distance in front, knees spread apart.

- Keep your trunk upright and hips and shoulders square, and lunge forward until your left knee is over your left foot. Feel the stretch at the front of your right hip.

- Hold for a count of 10 and repeat on the other side.

Note: If your front knee passes your foot, then move your front foot farther forward; your front knee should never go past the toes. Keep your trunk upright during this stretch.

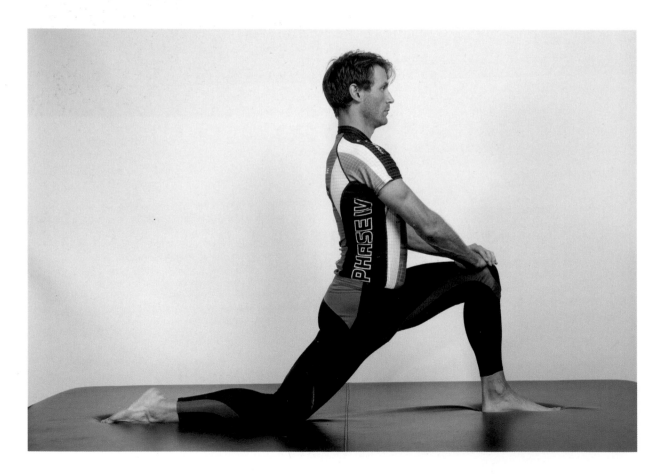

11. Standing Hamstring Stretch

It is critical to promote good flexibility in the hamstring muscles to maintain good running form and prevent injury to your knees, buttocks, and lower back. Notice that the model in the photo does not bend over and touch his toes because there is no need to stress the lower back.

Instructions:

- Stand with your feet pointing straight ahead.

- Put the heel of one leg up no higher than a surface.

- Think about pulling your buttocks back as you hinge at the hips. Keep your back flat as you angle your trunk forward at your hips. Keep your elevated foot relaxed. Stop when you feel the first sign of stretch in the hamstrings. Hold for a count of 10. Repeat on the other side. Do 2 reps on each side.

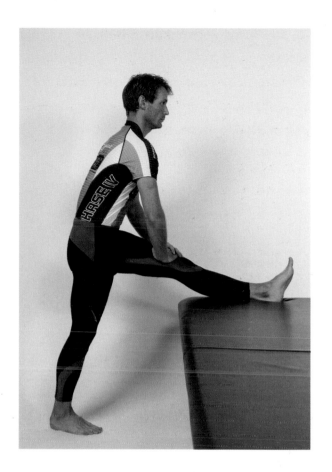

12. Standing Adductor Stretch

This stretch addresses the inner thigh muscle (adductors), a strong and powerful muscle group that is active in running. It both stabilizes your pelvis and moves your leg forward and backward during the running gait.

Instructions:

- From the hamstring stretch position, pivot your supporting foot, leg, and trunk outward 90 degrees and keep your toes pointing up as shown. In this posture, you should feel the stretch in the inner thingh.

- To get more of a stretch in your inner thigh, bend your supporting leg slightly. You can maximize a stretch in your inner thigh by bending your torso sideways toward the raised leg. Always maintain a flat plane from hips to head. Hold for a count of 10. Do 2 reps on each side.

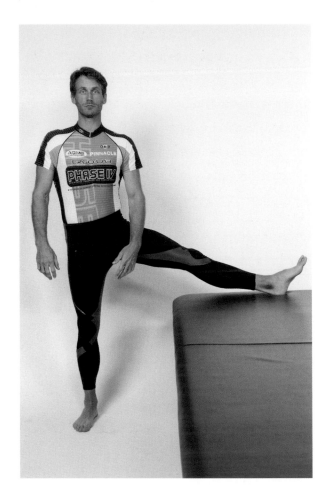

13. Standing Calf Stretch

Stretching the calf muscles is essential to maintaining the full range of motion of the ankle to ensure proper running mechanics and maintain the health of the Achilles tendon. Stretch the two heads of the gastrocnemius muscle by keeping the rear leg straight while leaning forward. The next exercise works the soleus, the deeper muscle.

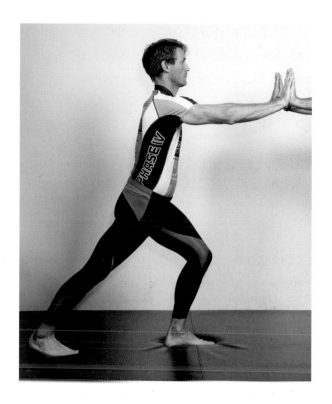

Instructions:

- Stand in front of a wall with a staggered stance. Keep both feet pointing forward and your heels on the ground.

- Place your hands on the wall and hold your back heel down as you bend your elbows to bring your chest toward the wall. The stretch should be at your upper calf.

- Hold for a count of 10. Do 2 reps on each side.

14. Standing Calf Stretch with Bent Leg

People often forget the soleus—and pay the price with shin splints and other deep calf injuries.

Instructions:

- In the standing calf position (see page 131), bring your back leg forward 3 to 4 inches (7.5 to 10 cm) and bend your back knee. The stretch should be in your lower calf and Achilles.

- Hold for a count of 10. Do 2 reps on each side.

Note: Oftentimes, this stretch will be more effective in shoes than when barefoot. Also, if you feel "jamming" in the front of the ankle, stop at the point where you feel it. Over time, that tension will subside and you should only feel the stretch in your lower calf.

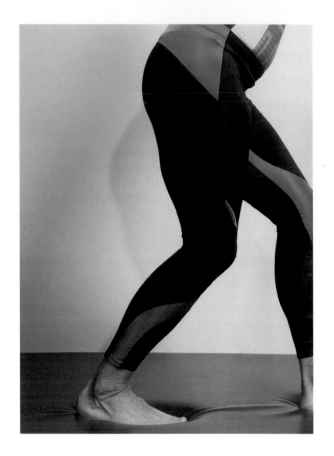

15. Chin Tuck

This simple exercise will not only improve your posture, but it may save your neck from the damage we all suffer with long hours of sitting. Feel the stretch anywhere from the base of your skull down into your upper back.

Instructions:

- Gently pull your head back, keeping it level. Your head should not tilt up or down. Keep your back straight and chest high.

- Make a double chin by pulling your chin in toward your neck. Do not bend your neck forward or drop your chin.

- Elongate or flatten your neck in back. Keep your head level.

- Hold for a count of 5. Perform 2 repetitions.

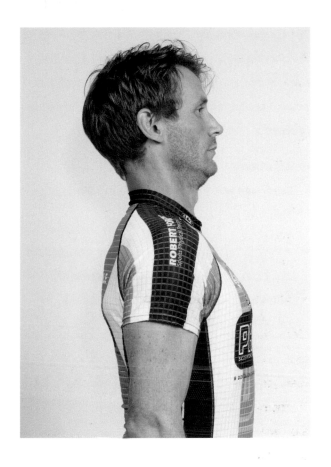

16. Cross Chest

This is one of several stretches that target the back of the shoulder, a problem area that is the source of rotator cuff injuries and other shoulder problems.

Instructions:

- Place your left arm in front of your body at chest height.

- With your left hand, pull your right arm across your body, holding the elbow. Keep your shoulder down and relaxed. Be cautious to not pull your arm down too hard. Keep your shoulders down and square.

- Hold for a count of 5 and repeat on the other side.

Note: If you feel a "pinch" in your shoulder, try to pull your arm first away from the body and then across.

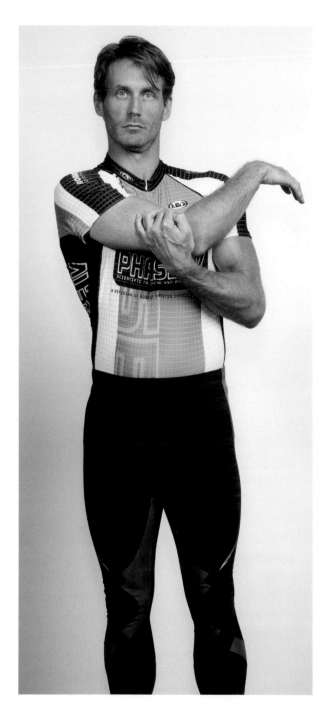

17. Standing Upper Trap

This stretch relieves much of the tension we all hold in our upper back and neck. It benefits running by allowing for the proper path of a vertical arm swing on the side of the body.

Instructions:

- Pull your left arm gently by the wrist with your right hand downward and to the right behind your back toward the right buttock.

- Bring your chin down to your chest and then rotate to the right to look toward your right armpit, keeping your head down. Feel the stretch from the left side of your neck into your upper back. Hold for a count of 5.

- To return, bring your head back to the middle position and then up.

- Repeat on the opposite side.

Note: Be cautious not to pull your arm down too hard during this stretch. Keep shoulders square.

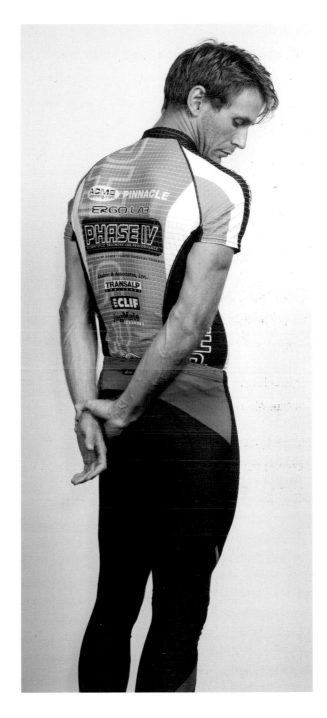

18. Penguin

This stretch was invented in our clinic to address the tightness we all suffer in the posterior muscles of the rotator cuff. It will improve the efficiency of your arm swing.

Instructions:

- Standing with head up and back and a "proud" chest, place the back of your fists at the pelvis (the top of your buttocks), with palms facing backward.

- Pull your elbows forward. Do not curl your shoulders forward. Keep your shoulders back. Feel a diffuse, general stretch in your shoulders. Hold for a count of 10.

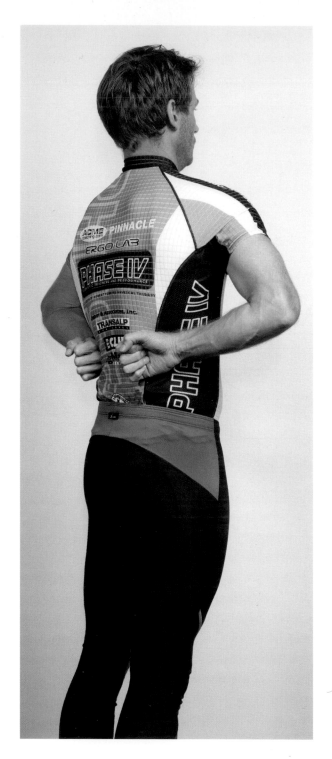

19. Pec Stretch

Most of us have overdeveloped, tight pecs that corrupt our posture, stress our neck, and deviate our arm swing in running. Tightness in the pecs prevents a good backswing and creates an inefficient cross-chest arm swing. This stretch restores that flexibility.

Instructions:

- Line your body up with a wall or door frame. Make a loose fist and place your hand thumb side at wall level with the top of your head.

- Take a step forward with the same-side leg to get a stretch at the front of your shoulder and chest. Keep your torso upright and your eyes looking forward. Keep your hips and shoulders perpendicular to the wall.

- Hold for a count of 10 and repeat on the other side.

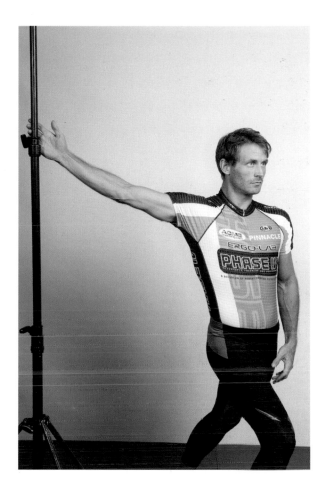

20. Overhead Triceps Stretch

The triceps muscle group crosses the shoulder and the elbow joint. Running will create tightness in this muscle group, which will corrupt your running mechanics and posture.

Instructions:

- Raise your right arm up overhead, bending your elbow so your hand is behind your neck.

- With your left arm, pull your right elbow back behind your head.

- Feel the stretch in the back of your left arm and along the side of your shoulder blade.

- Hold for a count of 10 and repeat for your left arm as well.

Note: Keep your head level and not forward. To get more stretch, side-bend your torso.

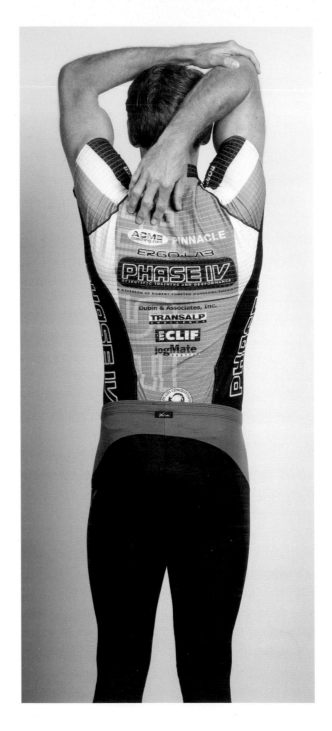

8 Strength Training for Runners

Why weights are a magic bullet for injury prevention, robust bones and muscles, and a time-saving shortcut to speed and endurance.

In 2013, Evan, a 25-year-old elite triathlete, came into the office complaining of one of the most common running injuries: chronic knee pain. It first appeared after longer runs and then progressed to pain during every run. Eventually, the knee hurt in daily activities, including going up stairs and during squatting motions. It had been bothering him for several weeks and was interfering with his training and his life.

There are many causes of knee pain in runners, but coaches and athletes have lumped them all together as "runner's knee."

Every injury is a puzzle that needs to be solved. To do so, physical therapists use two related approaches: a physical examination to find out which body part hurts (the damaged structure) and movement analysis to find why it hurts (usually a misalignment issue). Besides some sort of acute injury (which didn't apply in Evan's case), the misalignment is often due to a muscular imbalance—muscles on one side

of the body being stronger or weaker than the same muscles on the other side, and/or opposing muscles on one side of the same leg being relatively tighter than opposing muscles on the other side of the leg.

In Evan's case, the physical exam found the pain to be emanating from under the kneecap. This is caused when the backside of the kneecap tracks imprecisely in the groove between the condyles (humps) at the bottom of the femur (thigh bone). Because Evan continued running in that condition, he damaged the cartilage, the smooth coating on the ends of the bones, which doesn't heal easily, if at all.

The second step was movement analysis, and sure enough, during a video gait analysis of Evan's running mechanics, we immediately noticed that his form was off: His right knee was coming across the midline of his body. That was a deviation from normal running form, in which the knee should drive forward in a straight line.

Now, basic kinesiology (the study of movement) told us what to look for: something that was pulling his right leg to the left. We quickly assumed that was the right adductor, the large muscle on the inside of the thigh that moves the leg from a widespread stance to one in which the legs are parallel to one another.

For the adductor to overpull, it had to be either tighter or stronger compared to its opposing muscle group on the outside of the hip: the hip abductors, which draw the leg outward from the center when the leg is unweighted in the standing position. The hip abductors are made up of four muscles located in the buttocks region: the tensor fasciae latae, gluteus maximus, gluteus medius, and gluteus minimus, with the latter two doing the lion's share of the work.

With early testing establishing that the hip abductors were weak, the solution was clear: Stop the thigh bone from being pulled inward by stretching the adductors and strengthening the abductors.

After 3 days of doing strength exercises for the gluteus minimus and medius, and stretching the inner thigh, Evan was back on the track, running pain-free for the first time in 2 months. Just like that, the biomechanical deviation that caused his pain was gone. From that point on, we had Evan perform abductor exercises regularly as part of his health maintenance program. Evan began stretching and using the foam roller to make sure that his imbalance and knee pain did not return.

I love working on elite athletes, but not just because it's good for the ego. What I learn from them directly translates to treating regular people, who make up 99.9 percent of my practice. You see, the elites' bodies are so honed and fine-tuned that they respond quickly to therapy, getting almost instant results. As such, they become a learning laboratory for clinicians like me, teaching guides for the procedures I'll use on average folks, who respond to therapy slower. The same results I get from an elite athlete in 3 days may take 3 weeks with the general public. But the elite's experience gives me the confidence that what we are doing will work, even when the patient does not see immediate results in the first few sessions.

The Benefits of Strength: Speed, Endurance, Injury Prevention, Fat Loss, and Robust Muscles, Bones, and Connective Tissue

The solution to Evan's knee injury illustrates the tremendous power of weight training to effect significant changes in the body and quickly get results. Weight training allows athletes to perform much more concentrated work in training throughout the season. Strength work is incredibly time efficient; the three 15-minute sessions we're recommending per week in this chapter will recoup any lost running time many times over. Once you adapt to the rigors of weight training, your ability to perform work is elevated, your mechanics improve, your aerobic performance is enhanced, and your resistance to injury is greatly increased. Although endurance training alone increases performance, it is clear to us in our work with runners that supplementing with weight training results in larger gains than endurance training alone.

In general terms, weight training improves two muscle functions: propulsion and stabilization. It also can strengthen other structures, such as bones and connective tissues, making them more injury resistant. Here's an overview of the great benefits of weight training for runners.

1. Strength training turbocharges performance.

It's hard to get runners to listen when you tell them that they should lift weights to prevent injuries (unless they're already hurt). But if I tell them it'll make them faster and give them better endurance—and do it in a hurry—it gets their attention! So listen up:

Progressive resistance training gives you the Holy Grail of speed: the ability to generate more power, optimize running mechanics, improve your strength-to-weight ratio, and make your muscles more resistant to fatigue.

Strength training works by tapping the basic principle of fitness: To elicit a bigger response, you must do more work (i.e., create more stress) in the same period of time. Strength training provides a concentrated stimulus that can build muscular strength and power in a way that regular running can't. That means that what you can do in 10 miles in running shoes, you can often do in 3 sets of 20 reps in the weight room in terms of improving strength.

The goal of strength training, which is increasing the amount of force generated by each of the individual muscle fibers, translates into increased speed as well as greater endurance. That's because having more powerful muscles delays fatigue.

You see, the body is smart about the way it uses your muscle fibers to get work done. It only uses what it needs to, and no more. So as you make each muscle fiber stronger, fewer of them are needed to maintain a given running pace. Technically, the way it works is that muscle fibers contract in specific recruitment patterns to generate force. While the first set of fibers bear the burden of the workload, others rest, waiting to be called upon later. By increasing each individual fiber's strength, you use fewer of them as you run, saving some fresh fibers for later.

ROMAN CALF RAISE

Progressive resistance training is a central principle used for all strength-training programs dating back to at least the Roman Empire. Roman gladiators in training would do lifting exercises with a young calf. As the calf grew over time, so did the gladiator's strength. By slowly increasing the load we lift in our weight training over the course of weeks and months, we allow for physiological adaptation to occur and we end up with stronger muscles, tendons, ligaments, and bones.

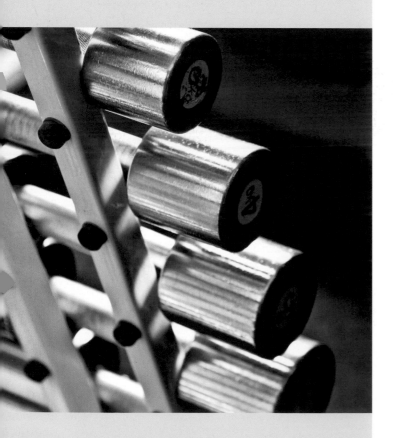

So in theory, if you use weight training to make your muscles 10 percent stronger, you can use 10 percent fewer fibers to maintain the same speed, and then you can use those fibers to keep you from slowing down in the last miles of a race. This is how strength training improves endurance.

With a program designed around progressive increases in weight, following the Periodization model, strength training will continually improve your strength and your endurance.

2. Weight training strengthens weak points to perfect mechanics.

You may be wondering why the hip stabilizers of a world-class runner such as Evan got weak in the first place, given his high level of daily training. But his experience is not unusual. In our modern, sedentary world, many of our muscles are unused most of the time, and those that don't get worked deteriorate. So it should come as no surprise that, in a sitting-based culture that lacks much hip rotation and side-to-side motion, we tend to suffer tight hip flexors; corrupted, kyphotic postures; and withered gluteus medius, minimus, and maximus. Sitting robs us of the hip strength and movement of our ancestors, which made them natural runners.

What does surprise athletes is that these muscles don't get worked much by "linear" activities such as running and cycling, which have us moving forward in one direction with no lateral motion. As a result, even elite runners are often too weak, imbalanced, and unstable to pull off all the natural economy of motion built into our bodies, leading to less than optimal form and injuries.

Unless you play a lot of tennis and basketball—activities that require lots of side-to-side motion—the only way to work the abductors is weight training.

3. Weight training maintains robust tendons, ligaments, fascia, and bones.

As with muscles, sedentary lifestyles neglect connective tissues and bones, leaving them too weak to tolerate the stress they are subject to in running. While strengthening your muscles, your weight training will also strengthen your tendons, ligaments, and fascia, the body parts of endurance athletes that are most subject to injury. Tendonitis, plantar fasciitis, Achilles tendonosis, and hip flexor strains are all common connective tissue injuries that too often sideline runners. These collagen-fiber connective tissues continually go through a breakdown-rebuild cycle that creates more or less strength in direct relationship to the stress placed on the tissue as they remodel themselves for performance. These tissues are hardened against injury at an accelerated rate with resistance training. Some of my Olympic athletes dubbed their weight work "Kevlar training" for its ability to seemingly bulletproof them against injury.

When it comes to strong bones, runners can't get cocky. Having heard that hard-core cyclists are subject to osteoporosis because of their activity's lack of weight-bearing stimulus, runners often pat themselves on the back, thinking that running naturally creates strong bones. But the illusion of runners' bulletproof bone density is shattered by the sport's fairly high incidence of stress fractures. A crack in a bone means that your exercise program outpaced your bone's ability to adapt to the load (which is why you have to gradually work up to greater mileage). As the thin legs and birdlike upper bodies of many runners show, you need more than impact to maintain solid bones. You need a progressive weight-lifting program!

Again, it comes back to weight training's ability to concentrate a load on your tissues. The bigger the load you put on your muscles, the more you strengthen the tissues that transmit forces to your bones and maintain their alignment. That's because bones are living tissues that are continually building, breaking down, and rebuilding. They bend under the stress of running or a muscle pulling on them. And when they do, it makes them thirstier to drink in more calcium, bone's raw building-block material.

Aging adds substantially to the risk of bone thinning for older runners. Bone density naturally peaks around age 25, but through the build-rebuild process you can keep your bones strong

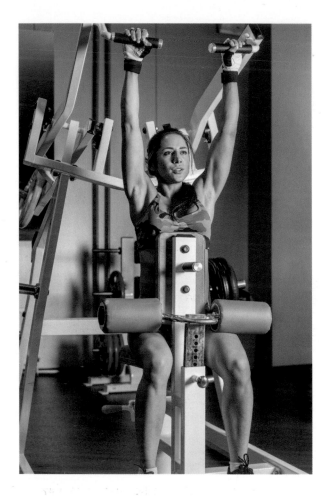

fighting bone loss. The more calcium you have in your bone bank, the more protection you have against bone thinning as you age. Start now, because you need good bones throughout your running career and your life.

Bottom line: All body tissues of an endurance athlete are subject to breakdown. Whether it is bone, tendon, ligament, or fascia, they are all strengthened and hardened against injuries at an accelerated rate with resistance training.

4. Weight training helps you maintain muscle mass as you age.

As with bone loss, muscle mass peaks in our mid-20s. Between the ages of 25 and 50, the average man loses about a fifth of a pound (91 g) of muscle every year. After 50, men lose up to a pound (455 g) of muscle a year! Because natural levels of testosterone and growth hormone plummet after 50, this muscle loss, known as *sarcopenia*, has significant effects on health and function. With less muscle pulling on our bones, bones weaken faster and the risk of fracture increases. As muscle decreases, the calories burned all day also decrease, which results in later-life weight gain. Done right, weight training will maintain muscle mass and maintain higher testosterone levels in later life.

by lifting weights. Two out of four women will suffer an osteoporotic fracture in their lifetime; one of every four men will, too. The mortality rate for seniors, post-fracture, is very high. The strategy for avoiding the thinning, fragile bones that put you on the fast track to osteoporosis is clear: Get proper nutrients in your diet (such as calcium, which is raided from bones in large quantities during exercise as an electrolyte from your sweat glands) and perform hard physical activity, the most effective of which is resistance training. It is never too early to start

5. Weight training cuts body fat.

The increased testosterone levels associated with weight training (in women as well as men) combine with the higher daily calorie-burn rate of well-trained muscle to reduce body fat—a huge boon for your power-to-weight ratio. Not only will slimmed-down, strength-trained runners now go faster, but they'll recover better because of increased T levels. Testosterone promotes recovery, especially when paired with adequate rest.

The Runner's Dozen: Twelve Essential Joint-Stability Exercises

Progressive strength training for runners could be—and should be—an entire book. (Get back with us on that one.) To be truly progressive, strength training must be timed to your running race schedule and Periodized—that is, coordinated with your run training to peak your fitness for key races. Early in your training cycle, when you are logging long, slow, flat miles to build your metabolic infrastructure, your weight training should be designed to simultaneously build a base of structural integrity and health.

Once you have developed a metabolic and structural fitness foundation, and before you begin any hill running or speed training, you should progress to pushing heavy weights in the gym—but only after this initial joint preparation phase. Because we don't have space to lay out the full strength program here, we have included only the first, and most important, phase of strength training: joint stability training. This simple but proven program will create efficient running mechanics and protect against injury, two keys to injury-free peak performance.

By first performing exercises that isolate the smaller, weaker muscles and tendons surrounding each joint, we create functional joint stability—joints that have the flexibility and strength to maintain good alignment through their full range of motion. This helps ensure sound running mechanics and injury prevention and protects your joints if you move on to the heavier compound or multi-joint exercises that we all know so well: hamstring curl, lat pull-down, squat, and so on. Along with the stretching exercises, this program is designed to strengthen joint structures so that all the muscles, tendons, and ligaments surrounding the joint will function in harmonic balance, keep the bones properly aligned, and keep you injury-free.

Eventually, for best effect, you should be pushing heavy weights in the gym, but only after you establish joint stability and correct joint alignment with the workout illustrated below.

In this first phase of strength training, we will begin the strengthening process with all-body exercises performed with ankle weights and dumbbells. Since the last thing a runner needs is heavy, bulky muscles, which would negatively affect the power-to-body-weight ratio that is the goal of strength work, we've designed the program to make you stronger and not necessarily bigger. This is not body building.

My strengthening program has a built-in bias to strengthen the vulnerabilities of the modern-day human body. After almost four decades of treating athletes, patterns of how a runner, cyclist, or swimmer is going to get hurt become quite clear. The human body has predictable weak points—so we know where it's going to break down, we can address these specifically in the strength program.

Functional joint stability is where strength and flexibility blend to allow bones to articulate properly throughout the full range of motion. Optimum joint function allows for more powerful movements and prevents injuries. The goal of the twelve prescribed movements described here is to create joint stability in three critical areas of the body that must function properly for injury-free, high-performance running: the joints of the pelvis, core, and shoulder girdle.

The stability comes by challenging the muscles to work in diagonal patterns, which is how they operate in the real world. You must keep these three areas stable while you run; therefore, maintaining strict form is key. Pay close attention to the execution of each exercise. Some might look similar to other exercises you've seen or done, but the twelve here have been chosen and created to be most effective at correcting muscle imbalances, and improving performance, while eliminating inherently dangerous exercises.

I call them the Runner's Dozen—strength exercises distilled from all those I have encountered in the nearly four decades that I've spent studying weight-training programs from around the world. Each one has been handpicked to address the vulnerabilities of the running body. They have proven effective for everyone—from spine-injured tennis players such as Pete Sampras to healthy Olympians such as Jackie Joyner-Kersee.

WHY CORE STABILITY IS IMPORTANT

The joints and muscles of the pelvis and spinal column must provide a solid platform for the lower extremities to function properly throughout the running cycle. The spine-stabilization series of exercises in this chapter delivers it.

You hear a lot about the importance of the core, doing core work, and achieving core stability, but little about what all that actually means and why it's important, besides developing an awesome six-pack. Well, core stability is crucial to athletes and everyone else because it refers to midsection muscles that are strong enough to hold the joints of the pelvis and the inherently unstable spinal column steady when we move. From that solid base, the big leg, butt, and hip flexor muscles can work to create movement.

In their misguided focus on the exalted six-pack, fitness enthusiasts and their trainers tend to neglect the deeper and less visible muscles that do the actual work of stabilizing the core. As a result, most people not only work the wrong muscle (the rectus abdominis) for the wrong reason (to show off a six-pack), but also do so in ways that are counterproductive to the real purpose of a strong core: to protect the spine against injury while performing daily activities and athletic pursuits. This translates into too many people injuring themselves doing superhard core work that exposes the vulnerable spine and pelvic joints to injury.

Ultimately, when it comes to training the core muscles, it is not a question of how HARD we can work them, but how hard we NEED to work them so they can create a stable base and protect the spine during sport-specific movements.

Anatomy of a Stable Core

In anatomical terms, *core* refers to the joints of the pelvis and lumbar spine, including the hip joints, the sacroiliac joint, joints between the vertebrae, and all the muscles that stabilize these skeletal parts. This midsection, where the body's center of gravity is located, is where all human movement originates. The large, prime-mover muscles of the lower extremities (hamstrings, quads, hip flexors, adductors, and gluteus maximus) and the trunk (lats, paraspinals, and rectus abdominis) all attach to the spine and pelvis. Stability is achieved when the muscles in the abdomen engage simultaneously with the muscles in the back of the body to hold the otherwise flexible spinal joints steady, thereby providing a sturdy platform needed to allow the prime movers to do their job. Crunches alone will not achieve stability.

While we all need a strong core to protect the inherently unstable spine during simple daily activities such as bending, lifting, and sitting, runners need an even stronger core to create a solid anchor from which the prime movers contract and propel us forward. But there's a conundrum here: The joints of the spine are delicate and highly susceptible to wear and tear and acute injury. Most core workouts I see in gyms all over the world put undue stress on the spine with ill-conceived exercises that compress, torque, and twist it. That's why safety and performance get equal billing in my exercises.

For runners, a stable spine is the key to training the core for injury-free, peak performance. It allows the hip flexor muscles, which are attached to it, to contract and create the high knee position that is so critical to good running mechanics. You can do crunches and work the rectus abdominis for years and never achieve true core stability, because they only work the front of the abdomen and are the wrong muscles for stability. The main function of the rectus abdominis is to contort the trunk for sports such as gymnastics, diving, and wrestling. As runners we don't need or want our trunk to move a whole lot. Instead, we want a solid, stationary core for the legs to work like pistons in the up-and-down movement that is running.

An effective and safe core workout for runners focuses on stabilizing the spine by improving the function of the transverse abdominis muscle located deep below the more popular and identifiable rectus abdominis (six-pack) muscle. However, as stated previously, true core stability is only achieved when the muscles in the front and back of the abdomen contract simultaneously to hold the spine steady. The handpicked exercises in our spine-stabilization series train both the transverse abdominis muscle in front of the body and the multifidi muscle group, located deep in the spine, to contract simultaneously to stabilize the spine.

In addition, this workout isolates and strengthens two key muscles: the hip abductors, which work to steady the pelvis from energy-wasting side-to-side movement while running, and the adductors, which assist the back-and-forth movement of the thigh. Strengthening the large and often-neglected adductor muscle group is the secret weapon we used to help Bob Kersee's track and field athletes win forty-six Olympic medals.

The spine stabilization series of exercises gives you a simple yet sophisticated method of creating stability with handpicked exercises that remove the risk inherent in most core workouts. These exercises have been proven safe because they're the ones we use to fix spinal injuries such as bulging discs, compressed nerves, and arthritic joints. This program has been tolerated by everyone from our 7-year-old student athletes to 70-year-olds, and it's the same workout our Olympic gold medalists and mixed martial arts champions use to achieve elite performance. So they will work for you.

BASIC BASE-BUILDING STRENGTH EQUIPMENT

You don't need much to begin hardening your body against the stresses of running during the base-building phase of Periodization. Forget giant cable weight machines that take up a den. Lightweight dumbbells and ankle weights, both shown here, will work just fine.

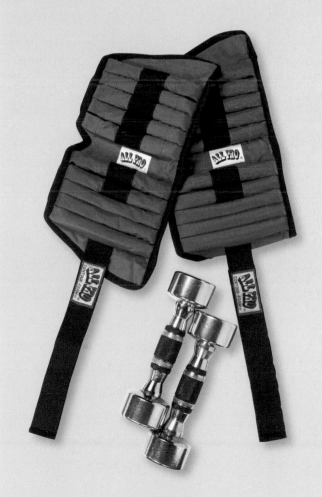

The Runner's Dozen: Rules

Perform this workout two or three times per week and always stretch before and after every workout. Follow the directions carefully. The workout is only effective if it is done with strict attention to the technique cues for each exercise. For the first three workouts, do the exercises only as directed. Before you start, keep these rules in mind:

- **Start unweighted:** No matter how fit or how strong you think your core is, start with no weights as you first train the neurological system to perform these exercises correctly.

- **Shift to 1:** After the first three workouts, add 1 pound (455 g) to your ankle and wrist.

- **Advance slowly:** Follow the directions on when to increase the weights and do not start the advanced exercises until week 3 or 4, and not before progressing to 2 pounds (910 g) on each extremity for all the basic exercises.

- **Top out at 5 pounds:** Progress by adding ½ to 1 pound (225 to 455 g) per week to a maximum of 5 pounds (2 kg). Never go higher than 5 pounds for any of these exercises. Using more than 5 pounds (2 kg) on each extremity is not necessary and only increases the chances that you will deviate from good form and negate the purpose of the workout.

- **Never work through pain.** If you experience pain, stop and perform the stretches for that area again. If pain persists, skip that exercise and try the others. Only continue if you can perform each exercise pain-free.

- **Inhale:** Before starting, perform 10 to 20 diaphragmatic breaths (see page 117) or until you feel ready to begin.

The Runner's Dozen

1. Bracing Maneuver

- Do this exercise for each of the spine stabilization series exercises. Lie on your back, knees bent, feet flat on the floor.

- Begin by making a sharp "psssst" sound. Notice how your abdomen and lower back tighten simultaneously and your back maintains a normal arch. This is a neutral spine.

- Hold this tension for 5 deep diaphragmatic breaths. Repeat 3 times.

2. Alternate Arms

- While lying on your back with knees bent and feet flat on the floor, make the "psssst" sound and perform the bracing maneuver as described previously. Hold this tension in your midsection and breathe.

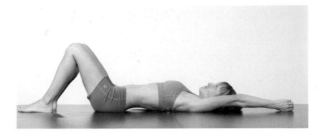

- Place your left arm on the mat beside your head with the elbow locked perfectly straight as pictured and your right arm at your side.

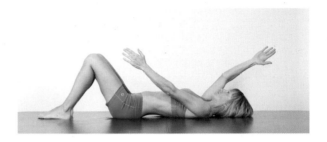

- Now, while holding the bracing maneuver, reverse the arm positions by moving your arms simultaneously at the very same instant.

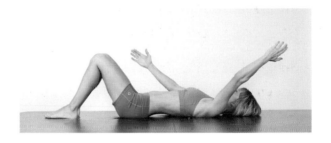

- Return to the start position; this is one repetition. Keep a slight (normal) arch in your lower back and pelvis still as you move your arms. Breathe. Maintain a neutral spine.

- Repeat 10 times and rest 30 seconds, then repeat 10 times. Only add weights as directed above.

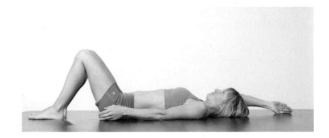

3. Alternate Arms with Knees at 90 Degrees

- Perform the bracing maneuver before lifting one leg at a time so the knees and hips are both flexed to 90 degrees as pictured.

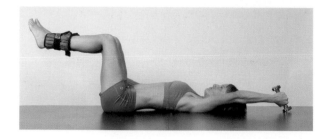

- Place your left arm on the mat beside your head, elbow locked, and your right arm at your side.

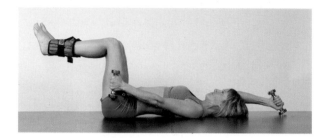

- Reverse your arm position while holding the brace and breathing and then return to the start position.

- Repeat 2 sets of 10 with a 30-second rest between sets. Only add weights as directed in the Runner's Dozen Rules on page 150.

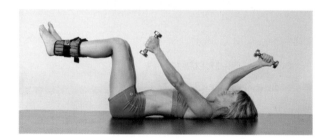

4. Dead Bug (advanced exercise)

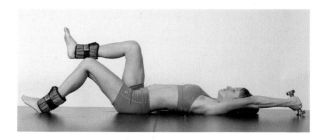

- When you begin this exercise you can eliminate exercise #2, Alternate Arms, but always warm up with exercise #3, Alternate Arms with Knees at 90 Degrees (page 152).

- To start, perform the bracing maneuver before placing your left arm on the mat beside your head and your right arm at your side.

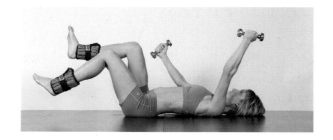

- While maintaining a neutral spine position with the bracing maneuver, lift your right leg to 90 degrees and keep your left knee bent with only the heel in contact with the ground.

- Now reverse your arm and leg positions by moving all extremities simultaneously. Pause for 1 count at the top and bottom but don't let your arms or heels rest on the ground.

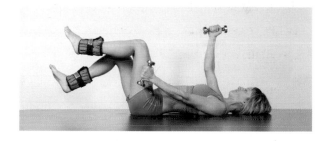

- Return to the start position; this is 1 repetition.

Note: During the exercise, keep your pelvis still and knees/legs locked at 90 degrees and elbows locked in the fully extended position as you move your arms and legs. Breathe. Do not pelvic tilt.

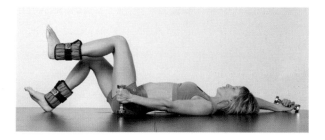

- Perform 10 repetitions, rest for 30 seconds, and perform a second set of repetitions.

- Only add weight as directed in the rules and never use more than 5 pounds on each extremity.

5. Abdominal Isometric (Partial Sit-Up)

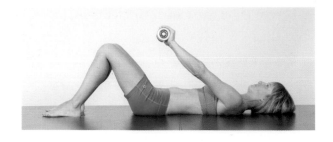

- Lie on your back, knees bent with feet flat, and your arms outstretched, pointing toward your knees. Do a pelvic tilt by contracting your abdominals and flattening your lower back down into the floor.

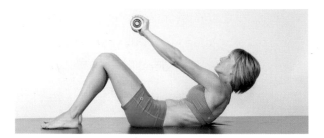

- While keeping your head and neck in line with your shoulders by performing a chin tuck, contract your abdominals and raise your shoulder blades up off the floor as you reach your hands toward your knees. Look directly at the ceiling, not at your knees. Do not grab your knees.

- Hold this position for a count of 5 and return to the starting position. Repeat 5 times with 2 diaphragmatic breaths between reps.

- Add 2 repetitions to each successive workout for a maximum of 10 repetitions. Increase holds from 5 to 8 and then 10 counts over the course of 2 weeks. Once you can do 10 reps 10 times, add a 2-pound (910-g) weight in your hands.

6. Hip Adduction with Shoulder Internal Rotation

- Lie on your side with your hips and shoulders stacked perpendicular to the floor.

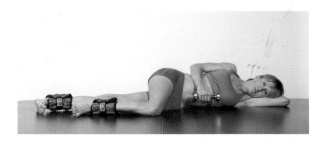

- Bend your top knee 90 degrees and lay it on the floor in front of your body. Straighten your bottom leg perfectly in line with your torso and lock that knee tight. Pull your toes up toward your head by dorsiflexing your ankle as shown. This locked knee and ankle position is called "locked and loaded."

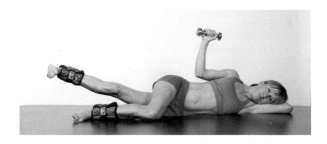

- Flex the elbow of your top arm to 90 degrees and let it drop in front of your abdomen, holding a 90-degree angle at the elbow.

- Tighten your abs while you simultaneously lift your entire bottom leg off the floor with the knee locked and rotate your top arm outward away from your body.

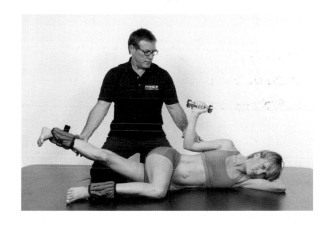

- Hold at the top for a count of 1 and return your arm and leg to the starting position. Repeat 10 times, rest for 30 seconds, and repeat for another set of 10.

Note: Be sure your bottom leg is absolutely straight and in line with your body and your knee and ankle are locked during the entire exercise.

- Switch to the other side and repeat the exercise.

7. Hip Abduction

- Lie on your side, supporting your head with your bottom arm. Bend your bottom knee 90 degrees as pictured. Tighten your abs and lock your top knee perfectly straight by contracting your quads while pulling your toes to your head. Hold the top leg exactly in line with your body. Look down and if you can see your extended knee, it is not in line with your body. Move it back.

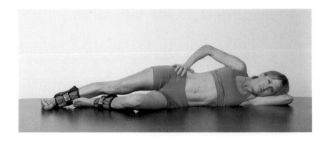

- Keeping your top leg in line with your trunk, place your top hand on your pelvis and push your hip forward. Make sure it doesn't rock backward. Lift your leg up, with your knee and ankle locked and in line with your trunk, so your foot is about 2 feet (61 cm) off the ground. Hold the position for 1 count and then slowly lower it back down.

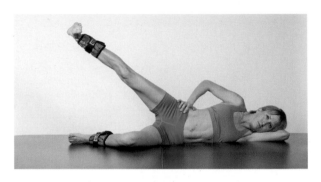

- Repeat 10 times and rest 30 seconds before doing a second set of 10 reps. Repeat on the other side. If you do this correctly, you should feel your muscles working on the side of your pelvis within the first 3 reps. If not, your upper hip is not rolled forward enough.

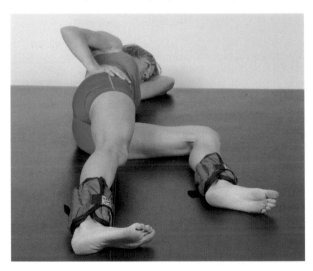

Notes: The hand pushing forward on your pelvis ensures that you don't rotate your pelvis backward and render the exercise useless. For this exercise to isolate and work the weak and neglected hip abductors, you must keep your pelvis directly on its side, perpendicular to the surface you're lying on. If you look down and can see your knee, move your leg backward and push forward on the right pelvis.

8. All-Fours Opposite Arm and Leg with Hamstring Curls

- Start on your hands and knees in the all-fours position with your hands directly below your shoulders and your knees spread wide right below your hips for a stable base.

- Tighten your abs and extend your left leg behind you with a straight knee and the big toe lightly touching the floor. Keep your back flat, hips level, and face looking down to the ground.

- Now, raise your right arm out to the side with your shoulder abducted 90 degrees away from your body, elbow bent 90 degrees, and palm facing backward as pictured. Keep your elbow lifted high and in line with your shoulder.

- Bend only your knee, moving your heel toward your buttocks as you rotate your shoulder and raise your hand to the ceiling. For the lower extremity, only your lower leg should move with each repetition, not your thigh. Your knee should not move in space as you lower your toe to touch the mat with the knee perfectly straight again. Repeat 10 times and then switch sides for two sets of 10 repetitions on each side.

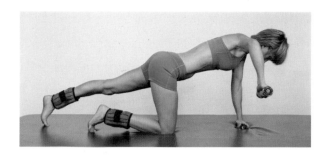

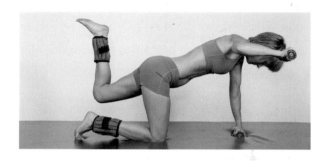

Note. Keep your knee straight when you touch the ground with each repetition. Maintain a stable trunk and level pelvis during the entire exercise. Avoid arching your back.

9. Front Plank

- Line up your body in the push-up position with your hands directly below your shoulders and your trunk held tight with a strong pelvic tilt (see top photo on page 159). Keep your buttocks down and in line with your body.

- Hold this position for a count of 5 and then lower your entire body to the floor.

- Repeat 5 times for the first 3 workouts. Progress to 8 repetitions for an 8 count for 3 workouts before progressing to 10 reps for 10 seconds.

9A. (Advanced Exercise) Front Plank with Opposite Arm and Leg Lift

- To start, perform a front plank (exercise 9) and hold for 10 seconds as a warm-up. Then lower yourself to the floor and rest for a count of 10.

- On the second repetition, steady yourself and carefully lift your right arm to a position next to your right ear (see middle photo on page 159) as you lift your left leg to the height of your pelvis. Repeat on the other side.

- Finally, lift your right arm and left leg simultaneously while keeping your pelvis and trunk in good alignment (see bottom photo on page 159).

- Hold this position for a count of 5 and repeat 5 times.

- Repeat on the opposite side.

- Over the course of 2 weeks, progress to 8 repetitions for a count of 8 and then to 10 repetitions for a count of 10.

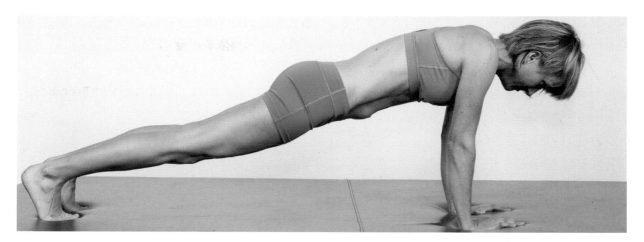

While doing a front plank, keep your hands under your shoulders, your trunk tight, and hold a strong pelvic tilt.

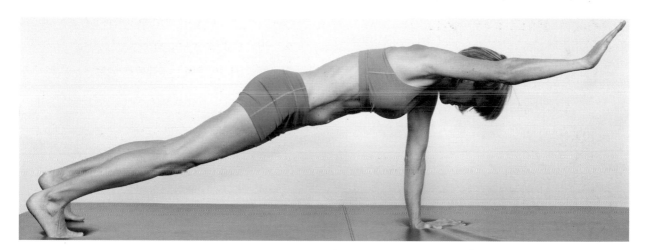

To begin an advanced plank, raise your arm to a position next to your ear.

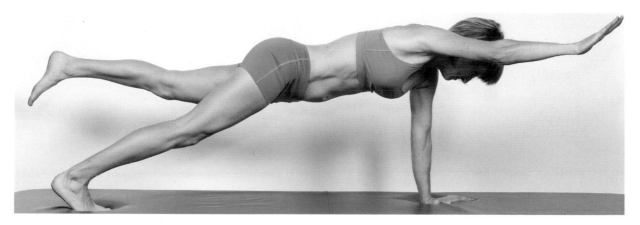

Progress to lifting your arm and the opposite side leg simultaneously.

10. Standing Squats

- Stand with your feet straight ahead, shoulder width apart. Bend your elbows 90 degrees with your hands at the opposite elbows as pictured. Keep your chest up and out and your head and neck back in line with your shoulders.

- Bend your knees and hips, lowering your torso backward. Keep your body weight over your heels so your kneecaps do not move in front of your toes. This protects your knees from injury (see the photo with the model standing against the board). Keep your back straight and your torso up and away from your thighs. Look down and check that your knees are spread right in line with your feet but not extended past your toes.

- Hold for a 5 count and raise yourself back up, pushing through your heels. Do 5 repetitions.

- Progress to 8 reps for an 8 count after 3 workouts and then 10 reps for a 10 count after 3 more workouts. You can then progress to holding weights in your hands in the same position.

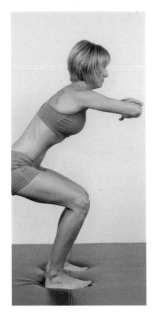

Proper alignment

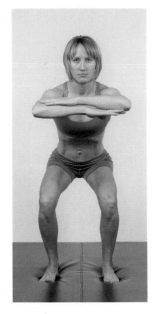

Proper alignment

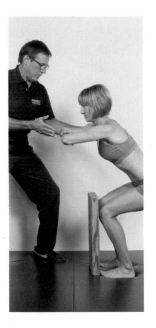

Proper squat technique requires that you sit back and don't let your knees move forward past your toes.

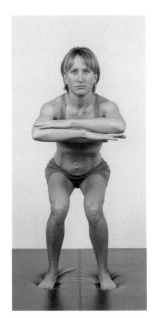

Poor knee alignment

11. Single-Leg Balance Rotation

- Stand on one leg with the other leg bent. Hold your arms with elbows flexed to 90 degrees as pictured.

- Rotate your torso to the right so your hands are pointing 45 degrees from the center. Hold for a count of 5 before returning to the center.

- Rotate to the left for a count of 5. Return to center.

- Put your leg down and rest as needed before repeating 5 times in each direction, keeping your knee in front of your body.

- Repeat on the other leg. To make it more difficult, perform this exercise with your eyes closed or on an unstable surface.

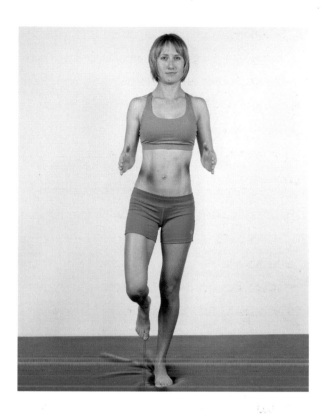

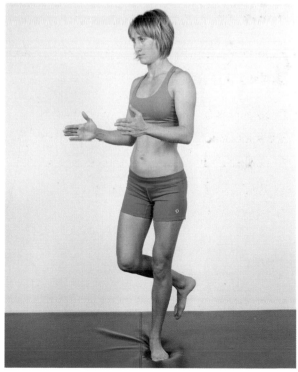

12. Single-Leg Squat and Reach

- Stand on your left leg with that knee bent in a single-leg squat and aligned directly over the foot but not extending past the toes. Bend your other knee and hold it off the floor.

- Hold your right arm abducted 90 degrees away from your body and the elbow bent to a right angle with your hand held high.

- Rotate to the left and reach across your midline for a point about knee high and return to the starting position. Repeat 5 times to each side.

- Progress to 8 reps when you are able and finally to 10 reps. Increase the benefit of the exercise by touching a point on the floor in front of your weight-bearing leg. When that gets easy, attempt this exercise with eyes closed for maximum benefit.

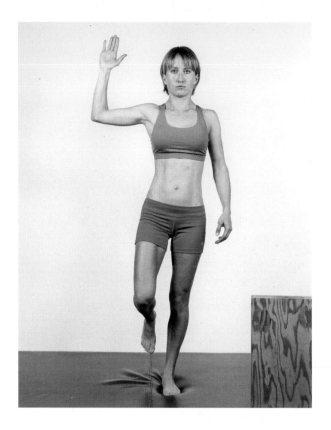

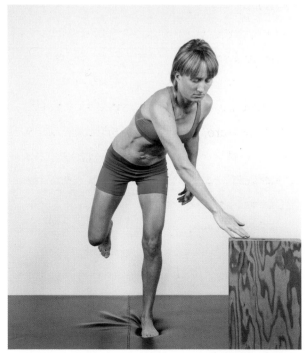

SECTION 2: Running's Big Five Injuries— and How to Fix Them for Good

9 Rehabbing Running Injuries

Use This Self-Guided Approach to Assess and Treat Running Injuries.

Ideally, after absorbing all the information in the preceding pages, you'll never get injured from running ever again or need a do-it-yourself guide. But stuff happens. Whether you find yourself reading this book because of the limitations of your insurance benefits, the high cost of clinical care, or because your local docs and PTs couldn't fix you up, the following self-guided rehabilitation approaches to common running injuries will come in handy.

Earlier in the book, I described how proper training methods promote the adaptations in physical infrastructure you need to be injury-free and reach peak fitness. In this chapter, you'll learn how things can go wrong with your body's repair mechanisms when you overtrain or suffer faulty joint mechanics and alignment issues.

The Anatomy of a Running Injury

Unless you fall down and break something, most of the injuries you're likely to suffer from running are overuse injuries related to the repetitive stress of running itself. Think about it: As you run, the joint mechanics are virtually the same for every step, with only minor variations in muscle and tendon function due to the pitch of the road. When joints function in the same limited motion mile after mile, there is a great potential for the stress to bear down on the "weak links" in your musculoskeletal system.

Unlike sports with more variation in movement patterns, such as tennis, basketball, or volleyball, where the stress is spread over different joints and muscles, running long distances can easily overload the same muscles, tendons, ligaments, or fascia in very characteristic locations.

The soft-tissue structures most commonly injured in runners include: the plantar fascia, (the thick band of connective tissue on the bottom of the foot that supports the arch); the Achilles tendons (where the calf muscles insert to the heel bone); the tendon-bone interface along the inside edge of the lower leg bone or tibia (causing shin splints); the hamstring muscles and their tendons in back of the thigh; and the iliotibial band (the broad band of fascia on the outside of the thigh extending from the pelvis to the lateral side of the knee).

TISSUE OVERLOAD AND THE REPAIR PROCESS

Every workout creates "micro-trauma" to the soft tissues and bones that make up the musculoskeletal system. Composed of structures primarily made of collagen, the body's soft-tissue system includes tendons, fascia, and ligaments. The bones that make up the skeletal system are made mostly of calcium.

After a workout, if a proper interval of recovery and rest is provided (typically 48 hours between challenging workouts), your body will repair the micro-trauma suffered under the stress of the workout and become stronger than it was before. Soft-tissue structures subject to stress are shored up by specialized cells that lay down more collagen fibers to strengthen the tissue. However, if you don't back off your training, allow recovery, or change your mechanics, the repair process eventually stalls. Instead of being rebuilt even stronger, your tissues are sabotaged by the relentless stress and by excess scar tissue (which creates additional dysfunction). This can lead to out-and-out tissue failure, such as a ruptured tendon, ligament, or fascia.

For bones, the process is similar. The body employs specialized cells to deposit more bone matrix in the most-stressed areas. Relentless training that shorts recovery can lead to stress fractures and even complete fractures.

With a proper training program and adequate recovery, the natural repair process—known as *supercompensation*—will gradually harden the body over time and enable you to work harder in the future. *Gradually* is the operative word here. To achieve injury-free, peak performance, you have to be patient. You can't push Mother Nature too hard. The safest way to gradually ramp up after an injury is through the walk/run protocol (see "Walk/Run Protocol: To Safely Start Running after an Injury, Go for a Walk," on page 166), which is featured in the injury rehabilitation grids in this chapter.

Two Causes of Overuse Injuries: Overtraining and Mechanical Imperfections

1. Overtraining: Turning Micro-trauma into Macro-trauma

You get injured when your workouts are too intense for your current fitness level or if you do too many challenging workouts in a short period of time without enough rest, or you do the same kind of workouts for more than 8 weeks at a time. The resulting micro-trauma doesn't have time to heal, so it progresses into a "macro-trauma." At that point, it's official: You are injured!

2. Mechanical: Watch Out for Leg-Length Discrepancies

If a wheel is out of alignment on your car, you're going to wear out a tire on one side faster than the other. The same thing goes for your body. An injury on one side only is a red flag, because a symmetrical body is subject to the same stresses on both sides. So if you have a mechanical flaw or asymmetry—you're bowlegged, have knock-knees, are an overpronator, have one particularly weak muscle group, or—the big one—have one leg longer than the other, you may find yourself injured regardless of whether you train perfectly or not. It may not show up for years or decades. But with enough mileage and age, with the repetitive nature of running, even small imperfections in your mechanics eventually will overstress some parts of your body until they break down.

To find the mechanical flaw that's causing the problem, you have to be a detective.

A good place to start is leg-length discrepancy. After 30 years of examining injured runners, I've found that the most common cause of unilateral injury and the vast majority of ALL running injuries is that one leg is either structurally longer or functionally longer than the other.

As noted previously, "structural" leg-length inequality may be created when either the thigh bone or shin bone of one leg is longer than the one on the other side. But this is rare. More common is "functional" leg-length discrepancy, caused by a torqued or rotated pelvis, in which one of the two large ilium bones that make up the pelvis is rotated and stuck either forward or backward. A forward-rotated ilium on one side in relation to the other will make that leg function as longer, while a backward-rotated ilium would draw the leg up and make it function like a short leg. Injuries can occur on the long or short leg.

The leg-length inequality will cause one of the two legs to function differently in an effort to even up the pelvis, so the spine will be held straight and the head in a level, neutral position. On the long leg, the arch of the foot is likely to be collapsed into greater pronation in an attempt to shorten that leg; on the short leg, the arch of the foot will be supinated (held up in a higher arch)

WALK/RUN PROTOCOL: TO SAFELY START RUNNING AFTER AN INJURY, GO FOR A WALK

Before you run, you walk. That goes for most things in life, including returning to running after any injury whose rehab should involve a conservative progression by time or mileage. You need to take it slow because, after injury, de-conditioning and loss of fitness are very rapid. In this rusty state, an overzealous comeback will often result in re-injury or another injury without adequate time for adaptation.

Before starting a walk/run program, you must tolerate a 25-minute walk twice per week for two weeks. You should also have a gait analysis done by a physical therapist, who will pay attention to the following (in order):

- Proper shoes: They should control mechanics (i.e., pronation).

- Arm swing: Your arms should swing in a vertical motion at your sides.

- Knee raise: Ideally, you should raise your knees so your thigh forms at least a 45-degree angle with your trunk.

- Running cadence: Your steps per minute should be at 180 (30 steps every 10 seconds) or better for proper phasic muscle activity and foot and ankle mechanics.

RETURN TO RUNNING

Over the years, I've found that the following conservative program yields the best results and reduces injury setbacks.

Week 1: Two runs with two full days of rest in-between. Each run should include:

- Walking warm-up for 10 minutes

- 2x (run 3 minutes + walk 2 minutes)

- Walking cooldown for 5 minutes

Week 2: Two runs with at least one day's rest in-between. They should include:

- Walking warm-up for 10 minutes

- 3x (run 4 minutes + walk 2 minutes)

- Walking cooldown for 5 minutes

Week 3: Three runs with 48 hours recovery in-between. They should include:

- Walking warm-up for 5 minutes

- 3x (run 5 minutes + walk 2 minutes)

- Walking cooldown for 5 minutes

From this point forward, the warm-up and cooldown walks remain at 5 minutes. The walk in-between runs remains at 2 minutes, and the running intervals increase by 2 minutes every third run, with workouts three times per week.

When you progress to a workout of three daily 9-minute runs three times per week, you can then increase workouts to two 15-minute runs per session with a 2-minute walk in-between. After two of these workouts, you can do a straight 30-minute run with no walks in-between. From that point, increase your running time no more than 10 percent per week. Avoid hills and speed work until you are back to your pre-injury weekly mileage and continue to ice after each run up to that milestone and you will aid the adaptation of the injured tissues and help avoid re-injury. Continue to stretch for the rest of your life and keep doing the rehabilitation strength exercises for at least 5 months post-recovery to gain full protection against a relapse.

in an attempt to make that leg function longer in order to make both legs function the same.

The self-assessment in chapter 6 will help you determine whether the cause of your injury is a leg-length discrepancy. The stretching and strengthening programs in chapters 7 and 8 will address some causes of functional leg-length discrepancy and may even correct it. If that doesn't help you resolve this common dysfunction, visit a PT who has experience dealing with this issue.

Evaluation of Running Injuries

When running becomes painful, diagnosing the injured structure is easy because our bodies break down in very characteristic patterns. Finding the cause of your injury is not easy, however, because the mechanical problems behind the injury are often very distant from the pain. If you're going to try to cure your own injury, you have to act like a physical therapist and start with a careful assessment of the history of both the current injury and your past injury patterns.

To flush out the mechanical cause of the injury, PTs will test strength, flexibility, and alignment. We look for the telltale signs of asymmetries, such as differences in joint alignment and function during standing, walking, and running.

For instance: When one leg is longer than the other, the foot of the long leg will usually be angled to the outside (i.e., externally rotated) because it becomes the easiest way to walk, as opposed to travelling over the toes. The arch on the long side will also be lower as the foot flattens out (pronates) to lower the pelvis on that side in an effort to even out the two legs and keep the spine straight and head level.

We also look for variation in callus formation from one foot to the other. Most often, the foot on the long side will show more callus on the inside edge of the big toe and/or ball of the foot. This is an indication that, while walking and running, you are pushing off more on the inner edge of the long-leg foot because it is more pronated than the short-side foot in an attempt to equalize leg length. In older and high-mileage runners, we even see bony changes on one side or the other that indicate one foot is functioning differently than the other, implicating a likely leg-length inequality. For instance, if the bunion (an enlarged first-toe knuckle) is present on one foot and not the other, this indicates a long leg. Once we determine whether the issue is structural or functional, we try to simultaneously treat the injury site and fix the mechanical cause as we progress through the rehab program.

Summary: Overuse injuries represent a failure of the body's normal housekeeping functions. After weeks, or in some cases months, of laying down scar tissue in an attempt to heal the micro-trauma caused by faulty mechanics and/or your excessive workouts, the scar tissue actually becomes part of the problem as the body's repair system ultimately fails. With overuse injuries, pain is the last component of the injury to show itself and with rest and intervention, the first aspect of the injury to disappear. When the pain abates, it does not mean the injured tissue has healed. Once the pain is gone, soft-tissue injuries still have a long way to go before they are fully resolved.

Self-Guided Treatment for Running Injuries Starts with the PRICE Protocol

Like everyone else, PTs love easy-to-remember acronyms that simplify the complex. That goes for the first phase of treatment for overuse injuries, which was historically guided by the RICE protocol—Rest, Ice, Compression, and Elevation. At Forster Physical Therapy, we added a P to the protocol for "protect." Injured runners must pay the PRICE of an injury by first Protecting the injured structure against further damage.

P FOR PROTECT AND PREVENT PAIN.

The first task in the rehab process is to protect the injured area from further damage. This is accomplished with the use of more supportive shoes, bracing, wrapping for daily activities, or correcting your joint mechanics/running technique, if you can run without pain. For some injuries, inserting heel lifts or orthotic devices in the shoes will limit or eliminate stress on the injured structure.

R FOR REST.

Above all, the critical first step in the rehabilitation process is to avoid any activity that causes pain. After all, you don't want to make the injury worse. Think about the way a cut on your skin heals; after a scrape or laceration, a scab forms. If you leave it alone, in 5 days the scab falls off and the skin underneath is healed. However, if in 3 days you catch the scab on your clothing and cause it to bleed again, it's now going to be 7 days until the injury has healed. The same goes for running injuries. Continuing to do activities that cause pain will prolong the length of the healing process.

Similarly, if you purposely pick at a scab to see if the skin underneath has healed and cause it to bleed again, you increase the time it takes to heal completely. The same is true for running injuries; if you go out for even a short run to "test" whether your injury has healed and re-create the pain, you will extend the life of that injury. Instead of a hard, crusty scab, your injured internal connective tissues heal by laying down more collagen, and this scarring needs to mature to become a functional "patch" that returns the resiliency to that tissue. This takes time. Like a broken bone, there is a 6-week healing cycle for soft tissues as well.

I FOR ICE.

The application of ice is critical to address the inflammation, swelling, spasm, and pain that result when tissues are injured. In both acute and chronic overuse injuries, inflammation and pain cause the surrounding muscles to tighten, in an attempt to limit movement and more damage. Ice helps because it constricts blood vessels and sets in motion a series of events to halt and reverse the swelling and limits the collateral tissue death caused when the pressure from the swelling cuts off the circulation to otherwise healthy tissue.

In some parts of the body, the swelling may not be evident, but make no mistake, there is always inflammation and collection of fluids in the tissues surrounding injury. These inhibit muscle function, result in weakness and loss of flexibility, and become a major obstacle to your fastest possible return to running.

Note: A clinical treatment program uses therapeutic ultrasound, electrical stimulation, and icing to address the pain and inflammation. Of these, it's important that your self-guided rehab includes liberal use of icing, whether you think it helps or not. If you want your injury to resolve as fast as possible, icing three times per day with ice cubes and water in a bag (gel packs are not effective) is imperative. Injured runners who religiously ice throughout the rehab program heal more quickly.

C FOR COMPRESSION.

Compression refers to the applying of pressure on the tissues at injury sites with wraps, sleeves, or braces, and is important in managing acute and chronic overuse injuries. When tissues become damaged, dysfunctional with scar tissue, and chronically inflamed, cells migrate to the area to clean up and then repair the injury. That sounds great, but there's a downside— swelling (also called edema), which is the body's attempt to maintain a fluid balance inside and outside the blood vessels by moving fluid out of them and into the injured area. Because swelling exerts excessive pressure on adjacent blood vessels, cutting off circulation and damaging otherwise healthy cells close to the injury, it must be controlled to limit the dysfunction and hasten recovery time.

The solution: Reduce swelling with frequent icing and compression, which work individually, but better together. Ice constricts blood vessels and sucks fluids out of the tissues, while compression physically squeezes the fluids out of the tissues, to be reabsorbed by blood and lymph vessels. The compressive forces should always funnel fluids back toward the heart.

E FOR ELEVATION.

Swelling can also be reduced by elevating the injured body part above the heart. That reduces fluid pooling and tissue pressure at the injury site by draining it back into the circulatory system. Lie down and elevate your leg above your trunk, preferably while icing with compression, to negate gravity's effect on the escaped fluids. If lying down isn't possible, sit with your leg propped at hip level.

SELF-GUIDED REHABILITATION: GETTING ACTIVE

Gentle mobility exercises in the pain-free range of motion are used to maintain and improve soft-tissue extensibility and help create a more functional scarring of the healing tissue while not aggravating the injury.

Once the pain is controlled, specific cross-fiber friction massage techniques are performed to break up dysfunctional scarring that has resulted from the body's repeated attempts to heal the injured tissue over time. You can accomplish this goal to some degree with use of a foam roller (see "Foam-Roller Protocol for Recovery, Injury Prevention, and Rehab" on page 172).

Once pain during simple daily activities and active range of motion exercise has abated completely, more aggressive stretching exercises are used to improve range of motion and start to address longer-term flexibility issues that may have contributed to your injury in the first place. Also, isometric strength exercises are performed to begin restrengthening the muscles surrounding the injury. However, all these exercises must be done without producing pain at the injury site. If you have pain during the exercises, adjust your position and/or limit the intervals of that exercise to eliminate it. Likewise, if you have more pain after the rehab exercises, you are doing them too aggressively and need to adjust accordingly. Only after the pain disappears during all of your activities of daily living (walking, squatting, pivoting, transfers from chair to standing or standing to bed, etc.) can more aggressive strength and flexibility exercises begin along with low-intensity cross-training workouts such as riding a stationary bike, running in water, or doing elliptical workouts. Although these workouts are important to maintain or reestablish aerobic conditioning before getting back to sports training, they, too, have to be pain-free or you risk setting yourself back in the rehab process. It's not acceptable if there is pain at the beginning of the exercise and then it disappears. There should be no pain during or after rehab exercises.

The return to running must be carefully orchestrated. Once the injury has healed completely, pay close attention to regaining full flexibility and strength in the joints surrounding the injury site as well as correcting the mechanical cause of the injury.

HOW TO USE THE INJURY REHABILITATION MATRICES TO REHABILITATE YOUR RUNNING INJURIES

The Injury Rehabilitation Matrixes in this chapter will direct you through the appropriate steps in the rehab process for your level of injury. To get started, read the left-hand column to find your "level of pain and dysfunction." By rating your symptoms during the activity listed, you can determine the extent and severity of your injury and set yourself on a path to recovery. You need to be honest with yourself about the pain you experience during the listed activities, and if in doubt, be conservative and begin at the highest level that describes your limitations. Once you have determined your level of pain and dysfunction (e.g., 1, 2, 3, or 4), follow across the grid horizontally from left to right, perform all the rehab tasks as prescribed, and follow the directives for a healthy resolution of your injury and avoid the frustrating injury-reinjury cycle! If you are diligent, you can be back to pain-free training in 3 to 6 weeks.

Achilles Tendonitis: Anatomy and Function of the Achilles Tendon

The Achilles tendon is one of the most robust tendons in the body, and for good reason: Three relatively large and extremely strong muscles in the calf (the gastrocnemius, soleus, and plantaris) all attach to the back of the heel bone (calcaneus) via the Achilles, and the forces they generate during running and jumping are immense, among the biggest in the body.

That's why, despite the Achilles' robustness, it is still at risk for injury, and it behooves you not to abuse it with poor training habits, but rather protect it with regular stretching and calf strengthening. The fact is, all injuries to the

FOAM-ROLLER PROTOCOL FOR RECOVERY, INJURY PREVENTION, AND REHAB

Too effective and too inexpensive not to use, the prosaic foam roller both heals and supercharges!

It doesn't look like much—a cylinder of dense, closed-cell foam a couple of feet (61 cm) long and generally around 5 inches (12.5 cm) in diameter. (The fancy one pictured here is called the Rumble Roller with foam knobs.) But the simple, cheap foam roller is one of the most effective do-it-yourself recovery and injury-prevention tools an athlete can use. We sports PTs like to say that all work is futile if you don't get recovery. Well, the foam roller can give you recovery and a lot more—self-myofascial release, self-massaging, self-joint mobilization, and even postural alignment improvement. For all those reasons, even if you're not injured, regular use of it will enhance your performance.

A foam roller works by using your own body weight to give you many of the same benefits of sports massage, including the ability to restore sore, kinked-up, tight post-workout muscles, tendons, and fascia to their normal tone; speed their recovery by increasing blood flow, circulation, and range of motion; and prevent future injuries by breaking down soft tissue adhesions and scar tissue. The body-weight pressure on the semi-hard roller surface can have a dramatic impact under the surface of your skin. As you roll on, for example, your thigh, the weight of your body flattens and spreads out the muscle and tendon fibers and breaks up adhesions between them, as if it's ironing-out the wrinkled infrastructure and whisking away kinks and any junk that could become irritations and anchor points for future injuries. At the same time, it "milks" waste products from the muscles and the capillary beds in and around them.

Foam rollers can help lessen the pain of many injuries, such as IT band syndrome and shin splints. You can target almost any muscle group with it. Here are some basic rules for using a foam roller most effectively.

FOAM ROLLING RULES

1. Always stretch before rolling.

2. Maintain three points of contact with the ground and area on the roller.

3. Use your bodyweight to apply pressure to sore spots.

4. Roll from distal to proximal (bottom of limb to top).

5. To increase the pressure on the targeted tissue, simply apply more of your body weight to the roller.

6. Find a painful spot and spend more time until it releases and the pain dissipates. If the pain increases over a 10-second period, it means that you are putting too much pressure on the tissues. Decrease some of the pressure on this spot and try to roll it out again.

When you have completed foam rolling, you should feel better, not worse (rollers should never cause bruising). Also, avoid applying direct pressure to boney prominences. Use ice to assist improvement in recovery and injury rehab.

FOAM ROLLER POSITIONS—LOWER BODY

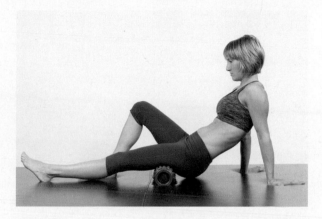

Hamstrings: Balancing on your hands with your hamstrings resting on the roller, roll from the bones at the bottom of the pelvis to the knee. To completely work the entire hamstring complex, experiment with your feet turned in, out, and pointing toward the ceiling. To increase loading, stack one leg on top of the other.

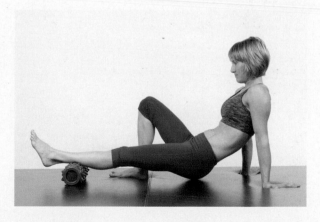

Calves: Balancing on your hands with your calves resting on the roller, roll from ankle to knee. Try it with your leg turned in, out, and pointing toward the ceiling.

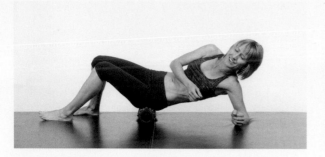

Piriformis: Sit on the foam roller, pivot your hips so that your weight is on your left buttock, and then roll forward and backward over your piriformis muscle.

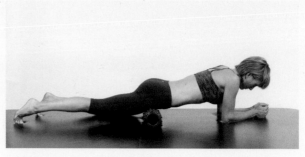

Hip flexors: Balance on your forearms with the roller positioned on the top of a thigh just below your pelvis. To get all portions of the small hip flexor muscles, shift the position of your pelvis, stacking the opposite leg on top to increase loading.

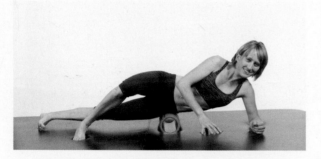

Gluteus medius and minimus: Lie on your side with the roller above the boney spot of your hip and below the pelvic crest, balancing your upper body weight by placing your elbow and hand on the floor. With your top leg in front of you for stability, rock your pelvis backward until you find the sore spot, and then roll forward and backward as well as upward and downward.

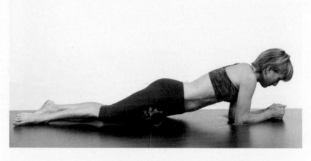

Adductors: With one of your inner thighs resting on the roller, and positioned at a 60-degree angle to the leg, roll from the top of your inner thigh to just above the knee. Balance on your forearms.

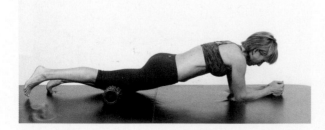

Quadriceps: Lying face-down with the roller on your thigh, roll from just above the knee up to your hip, using your forearms for balance. Try this with the thighs both internally and externally rotated. To do so, just shift the position of your pelvis to the right and then left.

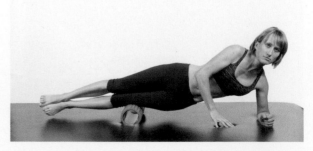

IT band: Lying on your side with the roller positioned just below the bony spot on your hip, roll all the way down the outer aspect of your leg to your knee. Stack the opposite leg on top to increase loading.

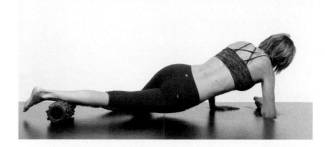

Anterior tibialis: Place the front of one shin on the foam roller, starting just below your knee. Roll from your upper shin to just above your ankle.

FOAM ROLLER POSITIONS—UPPER BODY

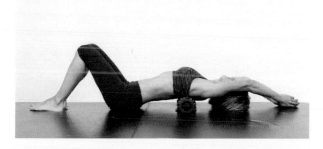

Thoracic mobilization: Start with the foam roller horizontal to your body and positioned at the top of your shoulder blades. With your fingers interlocked above your head and neck and elbows pushed inward so that they almost touch together, roll from the top of your shoulder blades to the low back and back again.

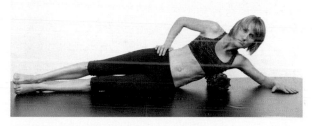

Latissimus dorsi: Lie on a horizontally positioned foam roll at your shoulder blade. Roll up and down to your armpit and just below your shoulder blade.

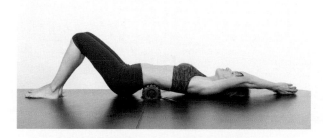

Low back distraction: Position the roller horizontally at the bottom of your spine above the sacrum and the two bony bumps. Have your knees bent up, and your feet, head, and upper back on the floor. Move your body downward so the roller moves up your back and then return to the starting position. Repeat twice only.

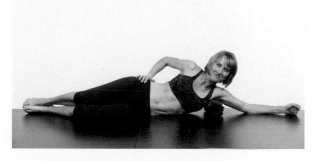

Teres major and infraspinatus: Position the foam roller at armpit level. Roll backward onto the outside of the shoulder blade and then up and down in a small range. Be very cautious if you have a history of shoulder dislocations. Once you find the sore spot, roll forward and backward over this spot.

Achilles hold the risk of complete tendon rupture—which Los Angeles Lakers fans witnessed firsthand in May 2013 when player Kobe Bryant suddenly was lost for the playoffs along with his team's hopes. As his untimely collapse on the hardwood demonstrated, the Achilles tendon sometimes suffers spontaneous rupture with no history of previous injury or pain. But more often, those huge forces manifest themselves much earlier with telltale pain.

To understand why the Achilles is particularly vulnerable to the stress of running, a short physiology lesson is in order. During flat-land, steady-state running, the calf muscles perform an "eccentric" contraction—that is, they lengthen in a controlled release of their contraction on the landing to stabilize the foot and slow down the forward progression of your body weight as the shin bone moves over the foot. Add the push-off that comes with acceleration or an uphill grade, and the calf now additionally performs a "concentric" contraction, which contracts and shortens the muscle.

The Achilles, being attached to the calf's three prime movers, is not only worked the entire time, but worked at G forces several times your body weight. Sure, it's designed to handle it—during a toe raise exercise, in which the calf muscles contract concentrically, an average untrained man can do it with 200 pounds on his shoulders and a well-trained man with more than 400 pounds. But that's a lot of stress on the Achilles and its constituent parts. Like other tendons in the body (but not all), the Achilles is encased in a sheath called a *paratenon* that produces a lubricating fluid designed to prevent friction. Heavy, excess movement and underlubrication (from poor warm-up, dehydration, or pure overuse) ramp up that friction, which you'll feel as pain.

HOW YOU FEEL THE PAIN

There are three different conditions of Achilles tendon dysfunction—Achilles tendonitis, Achilles paratenonitis, and Achilles tendonosis—and you feel similar pain signatures from each one. But with careful observation and palpation (what PTs call poking people and asking, "Does that hurt?"), we can make an exact diagnosis.

1. Achilles Tendonitis

The Achilles tendon, like all tendons, is composed of collagen fibers that are constantly reacting to the stress of the forces created during activities of daily life and exercise. In normal use, the body has no problem keeping up with the repair needs of fibers that get damaged (microtears) from the stresses of walking, running, and jumping. Achilles tendonitis occurs when the volume and intensity of these activities creates a stress load that outpaces the body's ability to repair the microdamaged fibers. Chronic inflammation results; pain soon follows.

Achilles tendonitis pain is provoked by high-exertion activities such as sprinting, running up hills, and jumping, but more moderate activities such as walking up stairs or even just walking will cause pain if you let it progress. Stiffness in the tendon may be present in the morning and after periods of inactivity. There may be increased soreness at the end of the day; often the pain is worse when you're barefoot and lessened when wearing a shoe with a slight heel.

You'll know it's Achilles tendonitis when the Achilles tendon is tender when you pinch it between your finger and thumb. Maybe, under close inspection, it's minimally swollen.

2. Achilles Paratenonitis (Sheath Inflammation)

Achilles paratenonitis is caused by an inflamed tendon that irritates the sheath (paratenon) as the tendon slides back and forth with muscle contractions. The pain associated with this condition is often exquisite and easy to recognize. It hurts when you perform any movements of the ankle, including simple range-of-motion exercises. Also, the whole length of the tendon is swollen and enlarged from the end of the calf muscle to the heel bone (as opposed to a bulbous swelling midtendon, as you will read about below) and acutely tender to relatively light palpation (finger pressing). In extreme cases, there exists an audible "crepitus" noise that feels like there is sand between the tendon

and its sheath. This indicates that a scar is forming between these two structures in reaction to inflammation of the tendon fibers.

3. Achilles Tendonosis

When the body's repair mechanisms fail to maintain the health of the tendon and the repair process fails, the inner substance of the tendon breaks down. This is a *tendonosis*, which appears as a firm, bulbous nodule about the size of a pea somewhere in the middle of the length of the Achilles tendon. Even after the acute swelling and pain go away, this nodule persists and creates more of an ache during and after activities. The nodule represents scar tissue surrounding the area of damaged collagen. If left untreated, it becomes the weak spot, vulnerable to complete rupture.

Note: Don't confuse tendonosis with heel bursitis (calcaneal bursitis), a condition characterized by pain and swelling at the back of the heel bone. It may be associated with inflammation of the Achilles tendon, but is a more recalcitrant condition that typically requires a comprehensive clinical approach to resolve. If you observe a swollen or enlarged bump at the back of the heel bone in one or both of your feet, you'll have to come in and see a guy like me for an evaluation.

THE CAUSE OF THE INJURY

Unless you hurt yourself by running too many hills, Achilles injuries in runners are almost always related to overpronation. Overpronation is defined by the degree the heel bone (calcaneus) angles inward toward the midline of the body during the stance or weight-bearing phase of the running gait. (See "What Is Overpronation?" on page 36.) Whether overpronation occurs in both feet due to inherent anatomy issues or only in the foot of the long leg (in an attempt to collapse that arch and "shorten" the long leg to match the short leg), an overpronated foot creates problems for the Achilles tendon in two ways:

First, the excessive inward inclination of the heel associated with overpronation creates an odd angle of pull for the Achilles at its attachment on the heel bone. Second, the corresponding instability of a pronated foot makes the calf muscle work extra hard to create stability.

As I mentioned earlier, the calf muscles function both concentrically and eccentrically during running. Of the two types of contractions, the eccentric (lengthening) contraction puts the most stress on the Achilles tendon. During the landing, the calf muscles work via the Achilles tendon in an eccentric contraction to slow down the forward progression of the shin bone, then switch to a concentric contraction to stabilize the foot and ankle and create the force needed to push off the ground. Overpronators have a problem because their heel bones remain too far tilted inward, meaning that the foot and

ankle are less stabilized and too flexible when it comes time to push off.

These two factors, a too-tilted heel bone and an unstable/too-flexible foot, cause the Achilles to struggle to pull up on the back of the heel bone and generate the right force needed for a good push-off.

REHABILITATION OF ACHILLES INJURIES

Rehabilitation of Achilles tendon injuries, like all injuries, is guided by the PRICE acronym previously outlined. As we like to say in PT land, "You must pay the PRICE of your injury to get better quickly and avoid chronic problems in the injury-reinjury cycle." Here, I'll apply the PRICE protocol specifically to rehabbing Achilles problems:

P for PROTECT: Because calf muscles and Achilles tendons are active almost all the time in daily life, take care of them by wearing shoes with good arch support, a sturdy heel counter, and a heel rise (which reduces the Achilles' need to stretch when you land during a running or walking step). When the Achilles tendon is injured, we advocate the elimination of barefoot activities, flat-soled shoes, and recommend heel lifts.

R for REST: Limit all activities of daily living and workouts that provoke any pain. Even if the pain minimizes after the tendon warms up with use, it doesn't mean the damage being done is minimized. To allow the body to begin to repair the damage, spare the tendon from further stress by replacing running with cross-training activities (e.g., stationary bike or elliptical machine) that cause no pain during or after the workout. Then begin slow running, per the walk/run protocol (see "Walk/Run Protocol: To Safely Start Running After an Injury, Go for a Walk" on page 166).

I for ICE: To control runaway inflammation and swelling, apply ice three to five times per day for 20 minutes. By controlling inflammation, you prevent Achilles tendonitis from becoming paratenonitis or tendonosis. You will also limit the amount of scar tissue that forms and shorten your recovery.

C for COMPRESSION: It is difficult to apply effective compression on the Achilles tendon because there's a risk of a wrap or strap irritating the sheath even more. Apply ice with compression three times per day.

E for ELEVATION: Elevating your leg above your hips or (better yet) above your heart is an effective strategy to control and reduce swelling in the Achilles. When done simultaneously with ice, it is even more beneficial.

SUMMARY

The first goal of Achilles tendon injury rehab is to control the early inflammation and swelling with the strategies of the PRICE protocol. This limits the loss of range of motion, muscle weakness, and scar tissue formation that will lengthen your rehabilitation program.

Secondary goals include regaining full range of motion, eliminating scar tissue, and re-strengthening the calf muscles that assist them during running.

As with all running injuries, a key is correcting your running gait mechanics, which will limit pronation and stress on the Achilles. If your Achilles issues are unilateral (on one side only), it strongly implicates a leg-length discrepancy that needs to be solved.

Finally, after the pain is gone, the stronger your calf muscles get, the less stress will be placed on the Achilles. Strengthen the calf to its full capacity with toe raises, with a gradual increase up to 1.5 times your body weight in your hands or on your shoulders. Proper running shoes and a scientific approach to your training that includes all the principles of Periodization will help minimize your chances of reinjury.

The use of heel lifts in your shoes, or wearing a shoe with more heel height, will take a significant amount of stress off the Achilles tendon by reducing the stretch on the Achilles when you walk or run. Heel lifts of $\frac{1}{8}$ to $\frac{1}{4}$ inch (3 to 6 mm) can be purchased at better national brand pharmacies. They must be worn in both shoes.

LEVEL OF PAIN AND DYSFUNCTION	LENGTH OF ACTIVE REHAB IN EACH LEVEL	ACTIVITY ALLOWED	FOLLOW PRICE (PROTECT, REST, ICE, COMPRESSION, ELEVATE)	STATIC STRETCHING
LEVEL 4 Pain with walking and active range of motion of the ankle. Also, pain and stiffness after sitting.	2 weeks, then move to Level 3 rehab.	· No running for 6 weeks, then begin Walk/Run Protocol (page 166). · 15 to 30 minutes of deep-water running or stationary cycling if not painful.	**P:** Insert ¼-inch (6 mm) heel lifts in both shoes. Wear all the time. No bare feet. **R:** No running for 6 weeks, then begin Walk/Run Protocol. **I:** 3x/day for 20 minutes whether or not it seems to help. **C:** When icing. **E:** Elevate with icing.	· All stretches in chapter 7 3x/day. Focus on Standing Calf Stretch and Standing Calf Stretch with Bent Leg (pages 131–132). · Use foam roller on calf muscle 2x-3x/day (page 173).
LEVEL 3 Considerable pain with walking or running. Pain-free active range of motion.	2 weeks, then move to Level 2 rehab.	· No running for 4 weeks, then begin Walk/Run Protocol (page 166). · 30 minutes of deep-water running, stationary bike, or elliptical machine every other day for 10 minutes/week.	**P:** Insert ¼-inch (6 mm) heel lifts in both shoes. Wear all the time. No bare feet. **R:** No running for 4 weeks, then begin Walk/Run Protocol. **I:** 3x/day for 20 minutes whether or not it seems to help. **C:** When icing. **E:** Elevate with icing.	· All stretches in chapter 7 3x/day. Focus on Standing Calf Stretch and Standing Calf Stretch with Bent Leg (pages 131–132). · Use foam roller on calf muscle 2x-3x/day (page 173).
LEVEL 2 Pain during or after running. Pain during or after hill running.	2 weeks, then move to Level 1 rehab.	· No running for 2 weeks. · 30 minutes of deep-water running, stationary bike, or elliptical every other day for 10 minutes/week.	**P:** Insert ¼-inch (6 mm) heel lifts in both shoes. Wear all the time. No bare feet. **R:** No running for 2 weeks. **I:** 3x/day for 20 minutes whether it seems to help or not. **C:** When icing. **E:** Elevate with Icing.	· All stretches in chapter 7 3x/day. Focus on Standing Calf Stretch and Standing Calf Stretch with Bent Leg (pages 131–132). · Use foam roller on calf muscle 2x-3x/day (page 173).
LEVEL 1 Pain only after running or speed work and hills.	3 weeks of rehab and reduced mileage.	· Continue cross-training as above. Flat nonaccelatory running only. · Cut daily running mileage by half. No speed work or hills.	**P:** Insert ¼-inch (6 mm) heel lifts in both shoes. Wear all the time. No bare feet. Remove heel lifts after return to full mileage with no pain. **R:** Cut daily running mileage by half. **I:** 3x/day for 20 minutes. **C:** When icing. **E:** Elevate with icing.	· Use foam roller on calf muscle (page 173). · Always stretch before and after every workout (Chapter 7).

ACTIVE RANGE OF MOTION	LIGHT RESISTANCE	MODERATE RESISTANCE	WEIGHTED EXERCISE	WALK/RUN
Warm up with active range of motion plantar flexion/dorsi flexion (like pushing on a gas pedal and bringing your foot back up), 3 sets of 20 reps, 2x/day. Do pain-free range of motion only. (This is used as a warm-up before the other exercises.)	· Perform Runner's Dozen strength exercises (page 150). · Rubberband plantar flexion (page 192), 3 sets of 20 reps 2x/day (if no pain).	If no pain, do double-legged toe raises (page 187), 3 sets of 20 reps 2x/day with no additional weight.	No additional weights.	No running for 6 weeks, then begin Walk/Run Protocol. No walking for exercise.
Warm up with active range of motion plantar flexion/dorsi flexion (like pushing on a gas pedal and bringing your foot back up), 3 sets of 20 reps, 2x/day. Do pain-free range of motion only. (This is used as a warm-up before the other exercises.)	Rubberband plantar flexion (page 192), 3 sets of 20 reps 2x/day (if no pain).	If no pain, do double-legged toe raises (page 187), 3 sets of 20 reps 2x/day with no additional weight. Progress to single-legged toe raises, 2 sets of 20 reps 2x/day.	No additional weights.	No running for 4 weeks, then begin Walk/Run Protocol. No walking for exercise.
Warm up with active range of motion plantar flexion/dorsi flexion (like pushing on a gas pedal and bringing your foot back up), 3 sets of 20 reps, 2x/day. Do pain-free range of motion only. (This is used as a warm-up before the other exercises.)	Rubberband plantar flexion (page 192), 3 sets of 20 reps 2x/day (if no pain).	If no pain, do double-legged toe raises (page 187), 3 sets of 20 reps 2x/day with no additional weight. Progress to single-legged toe raises, 2 sets of 20 reps 2x/day.	Toe raises with 10 lbs in each hand, 2 sets of 20 reps 3x/week.	After 2 weeks of rehab, return to running per Walk/Run Protocol.
Warm up with active range of motion plantar flexion/dorsi flexion (like pushing on a gas pedal and bringing your foot back up), 3 sets of 20 reps, 2x/day. Do pain-free range of motion only. (This is used as a warm-up before the other exercises.)	Rubberband plantar flexion (page 192), 3 sets of 20 reps 2x/day (if no pain).	If no pain, do double-legged toe raises (page 187), 3 sets of 20 reps 2x/day with no additional weight. Progress to single-legged toe raises, 2 sets of 20 reps 2x/day.	Add 10 to 15 lbs on shoulders, up to 1/2 your body weight; 2 sets of 20 reps 3x/week.	After 2 weeks of rehab, build mileage by 10% to 15% per week. No speed work or hills for 6 weeks.

Shin Splints: Anatomy and Function

The term *shin splints* is a catchall phrase that refers to nearly all pain in the lower leg except calf and Achilles tendon injuries. There are two types: anterior shin splints and medial shin splints.

Anterior shin splints appear as pain in the fleshy muscle in the front of the lower leg. Although this injury is common when runners first begin running after a layoff, it is rarely serious or persistent.

Medial shin splints (technically termed a *periostitis*), which appear on the inside border of the lower leg bone (tibia), are much worse. They occur from overpronation when you run too far too soon, straining tendons that attach to the tibia and pulling the periosteum, the paper-thin tissue covering of all bones, away from the shin bone.

A quick anatomy lesson may help explain what's happening here: Muscles deep in the back of the calf function to slow down the forward progression of the tibia over the foot in the stance phase of running. The tendons of these deep flexor muscles attach either directly to the medial border of the tibia or indirectly by way of tether-like structures. When they fatigue they begin to function poorly, the tendons become inflamed (tendonitis), and they pull the periosteum covering away from the bone and create acute pain (periostitis).

HOW YOU FEEL THE PAIN

Typically, shin-splint pain will first appear at the end of long runs or after extended efforts. Soon, the pain will appear earlier in the workout and sometimes abate as you warm up, only to return toward the end of the workout. As time goes on, the pain will spill over into walking and standing during activities of daily living. Occasionally, runners will pull up (stop due to pain) during workouts and racing with a complete fracture of the tibia.

HOW THE INJURY HAPPENS

The most common mechanical running error is overstriding. By definition, when you overstride you take too few steps per minute; therefore, your foot spends too much time in contact with the ground during each step. If you are an overpronator, this extended period on the ground (what we call the *stance phase)* allows the foot to pronate to a greater degree than it otherwise would with quicker steps. The result is that the deep flexor muscles of the calf remain engaged for just a few milliseconds too long each step. Mile after mile, this fatigues the muscles. As they begin to operate dysfunctionally, their tendons become damaged, and as they lose their elastic properties, they pull the periosteum off the bone.

REHABILITATION TECHNIQUES

In addition to treating the inflammation in the bones and the tendons with regular icing, it is imperative to break up the scar tissue and build up the muscles deep in the calf with foam roller work while progressing through the stretching and strengthening program, which is outlined in the Self-Diagnosis and Rehabilitation Matrix on pages 184–185.

However, the single most important factor for the resolution of this injury and to prevent reinjury is to increase your running cadence (i.e., increase the number of steps you take per minute). More steps per minute reduce the amount of time the muscles in the calf have to work each step and limit their load by limiting the degree of pronation. In addition, a light self-grip wrap around the shin bone will provide a compression force to help the periosteum readhere to the tibia bone.

If the pain is bilateral (i.e., in both legs), then the causative factors in the development of the shin splints are both overpronation and over-striding. If the pain is unilateral, then it is likely the painful side is the long leg, which is overpronating in an effort to even out your leg lengths during weight bearing. (See pages 98–100 to evaluate for a leg-length discrepancy.) This will have to be corrected to resolve the shin splint along with an increase in running cadence.

TOE CURL EXERCISES

These exercises are used in the Self-Diagnosis and Rehabilitation Matrixes in this chapter. Go to www.forsterpt.com and www.phase-iv. net for photos of the exercises.

1. Sit on the edge of a chair that has a small towel placed in front of it on the floor. Fold the towel in half lengthwise and stretch it out.

2. Place a 1- to 3-pound (.5 to 1.3-kg) weight at the far end of the towel and moisten the towel for better traction.

3. With your heel on the edge of the towel closest to you, crunch your toes and attempt to grip the towel and pull the weighted end of the towel to you. Once the towel bunches up under your arch, stop and smooth it out so the towel is flat under your foot and return to pulling the weight to you. Perform 1 to 3 repetitions. Increase repetitions and/or weight over time as you get stronger.

LEVEL OF PAIN AND DYSFUNCTION	LENGTH OF ACTIVE REHAB IN EACH LEVEL	ACTIVITY ALLOWED	FOLLOW PRICE (PROTECT, REST, ICE, COMPRESSION, ELEVATE)
LEVEL 4 · Pain on inside of shin at rest or with walking that causes you to limp. · Pain and limping after long runs and speed work. · Pain with walking after long periods on your feet or at the end of the day.	2 weeks, then move to Level 3 rehab.	· No running for 6 weeks, then begin Walk/Run Protocol (page 166). · 15 to 30 minutes of deep-water running or stationary cycling (if not painful).	**P:** Use self-grip tape to wrap shin or properly fit shin sleeve when weight bearing. No walking on bare feet. Wear supportive shoes in all daily activities. **R:** No running for 6 weeks, then begin Walk/Run Protocol. **I:** 3x/day for 20 minutes. **C:** With icing and as above. **E:** Elevate feet with icing and whenever possible.
LEVEL 3 · Pain on inside of shin during running, either at the start or end of run. · Pain after long run when wearing unsupportive shoes.	2 weeks, then move to Level 2 rehab.	· No running for 4 weeks, then begin Walk/Run Protocol (page 166). · 30 minutes of deep-water running or stationary bike every other day, 10 minutes per week.	**P:** Use self-grip tape to wrap shin or properly fit shin sleeve when weight bearing. No walking on bare feet. Wear supportive shoes in all daily activities. **R:** No running for 4 weeks, then begin Walk/Run Protocol. **I:** 3x/day for 20 minutes. **C:** With icing and as above. **E:** Elevate feet with icing and whenever possible.
LEVEL 2 · Pain at the start of running that warms up and becomes tolerable. · May have pain walking at end of day or in unsupportive shoes.	2 weeks, then move to Level 1 rehab.	· No running for 2 weeks, then begin Walk/Run Protocol (page 166). · 30 minutes of deep-water running or stationary bike. · You may substitute an elliptical trainer if tolerated with no pain during or after workout.	**P:** Use self-grip tape to wrap shin or properly fit shin sleeve when weight bearing. No walking in bare feet. Wear supportive shoes in all daily activities. **R:** No running for 2 weeks, then begin Walk/Run Protocol. **I:** 3x/day for 20 minutes. **C:** With icing and as above. **E:** Elevate feet with icing and whenever possible.
LEVEL 1 · Pain during palpation or when pressure is applied to the inside of your shin. · Noticeable stiffness in muscle next to inside of shin.	3 weeks of rehab and reduced mileage.	· Continue cross-training. · Flat, non-accelatory running only. Cut daily mileage in half. No speed work or hills.	**P:** Wear 1/4 inch (6 mm)-high heel lifts (page 179) in both shoes. No walking on bare feet. Remove heel lifts after return to full mileage with no pain. **R:** Cut daily mileage in half. **I:** 3x/day for 20 minutes whether it seems to help or not. **C:** Not needed. **E:** Elevate with icing.

STATIC STRETCHING	LIGHT RESISTANCE	MODERATE RESISTANCE	WEIGHTED EXERCISE	WALK/RUN
· All stretches in chapter 7 3x/day. Focus on Standing Calf Stretch and Standing Calf Stretch with Bent Leg (pages 131–132). · Use foam roller on calf muscles (page 173).	· Runner's Dozen strength exercises (page 150). · Rubber-band plantar flexion/dorsi flexion inversion/eversion, 3 sets of 20 reps 2x/day (page 192). · Toe curls, 5 reps 2x/day (page 183).	· Double-legged toe raises (page 187) with body weight, 3 sets of 20 reps 2x/day (if no pain). · No additional weight.	No additional weight.	· No running for 6 weeks, then begin Walk/Run Protocol. · No walking for exercise.
· All stretches in chapter 7 3x/day. Focus on Standing Calf Stretch and Standing Calf Stretch with Bent Leg (pages 131–132). · Use foam roller on calf muscles (page 173).	· Runner's Dozen strength exercises (page 150). · Rubber-band plantar flexion/dorsi flexion inversion/eversion, 3 sets of 20 reps 2x/day (page 192). · Toe curls, 5 reps 2x/day (page 183). Add 1 pound per week.	Double-legged toe raises (page 187) with body weight, 3 sets of 20 reps 2x/day (if no pain). Progress to single-legged toe raises (if no pain), 2 sets of 20 reps 2x/day.	Add 10 to 15 lbs on shoulders, up to half your body weight, for 2 sets of 20 reps, every other day.	· No running for 4 weeks, then begin Walk/Run Protocol. · No walking for exercise.
· All stretches in chapter 7 3x/day. Focus on Standing Calf Stretch and Standing Calf Stretch with Bent Leg (pages 131–132). · Use foam roller on calf muscles (page 173).	· Runner's Dozen strength exercises (page 150). · Rubber-band plantar flexion/dorsi flexion inversion/eversion, 3 sets of 20 reps 2x/day (page 192). · Toe curls, 5 reps 2x/day (page 183). Add 1 pound per week.	Double-legged toe raises (page 187), 3 sets of 20 reps 2x/day (if no pain). Progress to single-legged toe raises (if no pain), 2 sets of 20 reps 2x/day.	Add 10 to 15 lbs on shoulders, up to half your body weight, for 2 sets of 20 reps, every other day.	After 2 weeks of rehab, return to running per Walk/Run Protocol.
· All stretches in chapter 7 3x/day. Always stretch before and after every workout. · Use foam roller on calf muscles (page 173).	· Runner's Dozen strength exercises (page 150). · Rubber-band plantar flexion/dorsi flexion inversion/eversion, 3 sets of 20 reps 2x/day (page 192). · Toe curls, 5 reps 2x/day (page 183). Add 1 pound per week.	Double-legged toe raises (page 187), 3 sets of 20 reps 2x/day (if no pain). Progress to single-legged toe raises (if no pain), 2 sets of 20 reps 2x/day.	Add 10 to 15 lbs on shoulders, up to half your body weight, for 2 sets of 20 reps, every other day.	· After 2 weeks of rehab, build mileage by 10% to 15% per week. · No speed work or hills.

Plantar Fasciitis: Anatomy and Function of the Plantar Fascia

The plantar fascia is a tight band of dense connective tissue on the bottom of the foot extending from the heel to the base of the toes. When you move your body forward over a weight-bearing foot, the toes are extended and lifted upward, winding the plantar fascia taut like a skin over a drum. This action helps transform the foot from a flexible structure able to adapt to variations in the walking surface, to a rigid lever that supports the foot while it's on the ground, by limiting the degree that the arch collapses as the body moves forward over the foot.

HOW YOU FEEL THE PAIN

You feel plantar fasciitis as acute pain at the bottom of the heel. It typically occurs in one or both feet when taking the first few steps out of bed in the morning. Pain may improve or disappear after a few minutes of walking around the house, but will often reappear during the day after sitting for a while, and at the end of the day. Pain may be worse when barefoot or in shoes with poor arch support. The pain may also be present at the start of a running workout and improve as you warm up, which is NOT an indication that you can continue to run. In some cases, the pain may be more in the arch area.

Additionally, some runners will grow a bone spur off the heel where the plantar fascia attaches. Although this may prolong the rehabilitation process, it does not necessarily preclude you from resolving the injury and getting back to pain-free running.

HOW THE INJURY HAPPENS

The plantar fascia can be damaged in several ways. The least likely scenario is that it gets bruised and injured by a pointy rock or other obstacle in your path as you walk, hike, or run. This needs to be addressed with the same rehab procedures used for the more common mechanical cause of injury to this structure.

A very common cause of plantar fasciitis is overpronation, which overburdens the plantar fascia by leaving the foot in a flexible posture with the arch collapsed, just at the time in the running gait cycle when it should be supinated and rigid, which would allow for the efficient transfer of power from the leg to the ground during the push-off phase.

Finally, the most common cause of plantar fascia pain is leg-length discrepancy, which will often result in unilateral pain (i.e., pain in one foot and not the other). Leg-length discrepancy will cause one foot to pronate further than the other in an attempt to lower the arch and shorten the long leg to correct the leg-length inequality. (See pages 98–100 to evaluate for a leg-length discrepancy.)

REHABILITATION TECHNIQUES

Although plantar fasciitis can be one of the most recalcitrant running injuries if left untreated, a quick resolution can often be accomplished if you jump into rehab mode quickly, address the mechanical cause of the leg-length imbalance, and correct your running gait mechanics when you get back to your workouts. Local treatment with ice and the foam roller and addressing the mechanical cause must be conducted concurrently for this injury to resolve.

The use of heel lifts in both of your shoes, or wearing shoes with more heel height, will take a significant amount of stress off the plantar fascia. Heel lifts of ⅛ to ¼ inch (3 to 6 mm) can be purchased at better national brand pharmacies. They must be worn in both shoes.

TOE RAISES

DOUBLE-LEGGED TOE RAISE

These exercises are in the Self-Diagnosis and Rehabilitation Matrixes in this chapter. Go to www.forsterpt.com and www.phase-iv.net for photos of the exercises.

1. Warm up by doing both the straight-knee and bent-knee standing calf stretches (pages 131 and 132).

2. Stand with your feet hip-width apart, toes straight ahead, and knees straight.

3. Push through the ball of your foot and raise your heels off the ground as far as they can go without pain.

4. Lower yourself to the ground.

5. Do 10 to 20 repetitions. Rest for 30 seconds and repeat.

6. Finally, warm down by doing both the straight-knee and bent-knee standing calf stretches.

SINGLE-LEGGED TOE RAISE

1. Warm up with straight knee and bent knee standing calf stretches AND double-legged toe raises.

2. Stand with your feet hip-width apart. Bend your right knee and place the top of your right foot behind your left knee.

3. Now, balancing on your left foot, simply push through the ball of the left foot and raise your heel off of the floor.

4. Lower yourself slowly to the starting position and repeat. Do 10 to 20 repetitions, then repeat on the right foot. Do 2 sets of repetitions on each foot. Once this becomes easy, try it with your eyes closed.

LEVEL OF PAIN AND DYSFUNCTION	LENGTH OF ACTIVE REHAB IN EACH LEVEL	ACTIVITY ALLOWED	FOLLOW PRICE (PROTECT, REST, ICE, COMPRESSION, ELEVATE)
LEVEL 4 · Pain under heel is severe on your first steps out of bed. · Pain under heel is severe with extended standing and walking. · Pain under heel worse at end of long day on your feet.	2 weeks, then move to Level 3 rehab.	· No running for 6 weeks, then begin Walk/Run Protocol (page 166). · 15 to 30 minutes of deep-water running or stationary cycling if not painful.	**P:** Heel lifts (page 187). No bare feet. Wear supportive shoes. **R:** No running for 6 weeks, then begin walk/run protocol. **I:** 3x/day for 20 minutes whether it seems to help or not. **C:** With icing 3x/day. **E:** Elevate with icing.
LEVEL 3 · Pain severe on first steps out of bed. · Pain with extended standing and walking.	2 weeks, then move to Level 2 rehab.	· No running for 4 weeks, then begin Walk/Run Protocol (page 166). · 30 minutes of deep-water running or stationary bike every other day up to 10 minutes/week.	**P:** Heel lifts (page 187). No bare feet. Wear supportive shoes. **R:** No running for 4 weeks then begin walk/run protocol **I:** 3x/day for 20 minutes whether it seems to help or not. **C:** With icing 3x/day. **E:** Elevate with icing.
LEVEL 2 · Pain severe on first steps out of bed. · Pain running or after running.	2 weeks, then move to Level 1 rehab.	· No running for 2 weeks, then begin Walk/Run Protocol (page 166). · 30 minutes of deep-water running or stationary bike every other day up to 10 minutes per week.	**P:** Heel lifts (page 187). No bare feet. Wear supportive shoes. **R:** No running for 2 weeks then begin walk/run protocol **I:** 3x/day for 20 minutes whether it seems to help or not. **C:** With icing 3x/day. **E:** Elevate with icing.
LEVEL 1 Pain with extended runs/speed/hills, and high weekly mileage.	3 weeks of rehab and reduced mileage.	· Continue cross-training. · Flat non-accelatory running only. · Cut daily mileage by half. · No speed work or hills.	**P:** Heel lifts (page 187). No bare feet. Wear supportive shoes. **R:** Cut daily mileage by half **I:** 3x/day for 20 minutes whether it seems to help or not. **C:** With icing 3x/day. **E:** Elevate with icing.

STATIC STRETCHING	LIGHT RESISTANCE	MODERATE RESISTANCE	WEIGHTED EXERCISE	WALK/RUN
All stretches 3x/day. Focus on standing calf stretch in 2 positions (pages 131–132).	· Runner's Dozen strength exercises (page 150). · Rubber-band plantar flexion/dorsi flexion inversion/eversion, 3 sets of 20 reps 2x/day (page 192). · Toe curls, 5 reps 2x/day (page 183).	Double-legged toe raises with body weight only (page 187), 3 sets of 20 reps 2x/day (if no pain).	No additional weights.	· No running for 6 weeks, then begin Walk/Run Protocol. · No walking for exercise.
· All stretches 3x/day. Focus on standing calf stretch in 2 positions (pages 131–132). · Use foam roller on calf muscle (page 173).	· Runner's Dozen strength exercises (page 150). · Rubber-band plantar flexion/dorsi flexion inversion/eversion, 3 sets of 20 reps 2x/day (page 192). · Toe curls, 5 reps 2x/day (page 183).	Double-legged toe raises (page 187), 3 sets of 20 reps 2x/day. Progress to single-legged toe raises (if no pain)	No additional weights.	· No running for 4 weeks, then begin Walk/Run Protocol. · No walking for exercise.
· All stretches 3x/day. Focus on standing calf stretch in 2 positions (pages 131–132). · Use foam roller on calf muscle (page 173).	· Runner's Dozen strength exercises (page 150). · Rubber-band plantar flexion/dorsi flexion inversion/eversion, 3 sets of 20 reps 2x/day (page 192). · Toe curls, 5 reps 2x/day (page 183).	Double-legged toe raises (page 187), 3 sets of 20 reps 2x/day as a warm-up. Progress to single-legged toe raises.	· Toe raises with 10 lbs in each hand, 2 sets of 20 reps 2x/day. · Stretch before and after each session.	After 2 weeks of rehab return to running per Walk/Run Protocol.
· Always stretch before and after every workout. · Use foam roller on calf muscle (page 173).	· Runner's Dozen strength exercises (page 150). · Rubber-band plantar flexion/dorsi flexion inversion/eversion, 3 sets of 20 reps 2x/day (page 192). · Toe curls, 5 reps 2x/day (page 183).	Double-legged toe raises (page 187), 3 sets of 20 reps 2x/day. Progress to single-legged toe raises, 2 sets of 20 reps 2x/day as a warm-up.	· Toe raises with 20 lbs in each hand, 2 sets of 20 reps 3x/week. · Every week, add 10 to 15 lbs on shoulders, until you reach half your body weight.	· After 2 weeks of rehab, build mileage by 10% to 15% per week. · No speed work or hills.

Iliotibial (IT) Band Syndrome: Anatomy and Function of the IT Band

The IT band is a thick band of fascia that extends from the pelvis down along the outside of the thigh to below the knee, attaching on the outside of the lower leg bone (the tibia). The IT band functions to stabilize the thigh bone and knee during the weight-bearing "stance" phase of the running gait and helps guide the lower leg as it swings forward through the air in the "swing" phase.

Just before foot strike, the IT band slides over a bony prominence on the outside of the knee called the lateral epicondyle. An internal structure called a bursa (a fluid-filled sac that looks like a blister) prevents friction between the bony prominence and the IT band.

HOW YOU FEEL THE PAIN

Iliotibial band problems can occur at one end or the other: at the top, where it originates on the lateral side of the pelvis, or more commonly at the lower end, at the site of the bursa on the outside of the knee.

This lower IT band pain tends to appear suddenly on a run, and it often becomes so severe, you have to limp or stop the workout and walk home. Although it does not represent a high degree of damage to the bursa or the IT band itself, it can be one of the most painful conditions runners suffer. If you ignore the pain

and continue to run, the pain will progress to daily activities such as stair climbing, squatting, and pivoting.

At the top of the IT band, where it attaches to the outside of the pelvis bone (the ilium) and the surrounding muscles, the pain can come on more gradually. Although less intense up there, it can be equally persistent.

Pain in either the top or the bottom of the IT band should *not* be ignored. The problem can be very stubborn and difficult to resolve if you run through the pain for weeks or months.

DIFFERENTIAL DIAGNOSIS

Lateral knee pain can also represent a tendonitis of the popliteus muscle, which often accompanies IT band syndrome or can exist in isolation. Pain here can also be from a torn lateral meniscus, the cartilage disc between the thigh bone (femur) and the shin bone (tibia).

To determine whether your lateral knee pain involves the popliteus muscle-tendon complex, try to determine whether the pain is worse during downhill running, the telltale sign of a popliteus tendonitis. Also, if you feel pain and tightness at the very top of the calf on the outside edge, it may implicate this muscle as the injured structure. Symptoms of a lateral meniscus tear include clicking, locking, and buckling.

If you receive an injection for the IT band, and it does not reduce the pain even temporarily, then consider these possible diagnoses and seek treatment from an experienced physical therapist. Rehab for these conditions is beyond the scope of a self-help injury guide like this.

However, if your pain is at the top end of the IT band along the outside edge of the pelvis, which usually begins more gradually as a subtle ache that is worse at the end of the run and after longer runs, a do-it-yourself rehab, as outlined in the matrix (see pages 194–195), will most likely work to alleviate the pain.

HOW THE INJURY HAPPENS

If the lateral knee pain is symmetrical (i.e., it occurs bilaterally at the outside of both knees), it may be because you are somewhat bowlegged (technically, *genu varum*; see alignment evaluation on page 101). Bowleggedness places more stress on the IT bands, which have less clearance to slide past the bony prominence on the outside of a knee called the lateral epicondyle. Likewise, if the IT bands are tight, the bursa can easily become inflamed.

The most common cause of IT band syndrome is overpronation of the foot. When the foot overpronates, it causes excessive internal rotation of the lower leg bone late in the stance phase, which alters the angle of pull of the IT band and irritates the bursa. If the IT band pain is unilateral (i.e., only on one side), it might be that one foot is pronating more than the other as an adaptation for a long leg on that side (see page 99 regarding leg-length discrepancies).

With overpronation, the arch on that foot will collapse, essentially shortening the leg to lower that side of the pelvis and even up the leg-length inequality, which will keep the spine straight and the head level.

Since the lower end of the IT band moves back and forth when the knee bends and straightens with every step, and it hinges from its upper attachment at the pelvis, any deviation in alignment of the pelvis has the potential to change the angle or pull an IT band and create friction at the bursa as well. For instance, if there's any asymmetry between the two large ilium bones that make up the right and left side of the pelvis, it will alter the angle at which the band glides across the prominence at the outside of the knee and irritate the bursa.

Over time, the bursa becomes inflamed and swollen and causes even more impingement between the IT band and the lateral epicondyle. The pain is severe enough that it typically limits running before it can cause significant damage to the bursa or the IT band itself. However, if you respond to the pain by altering your gait in an effort to limit the pain, you are likely to cause excessive stress on other structures and cause additional, potentially more damaging injuries.

REHABILITATION PLAN

The primary approach to all IT band syndromes is to limit the amount of pronation in the foot when you run. And the best way to limit

RUBBER BAND ANKLE EXERCISE PROGRAM

Stretching a thick rubber band or rubber tubing can help stretch injured or at-risk muscles and joints. These exercises are in the Self-Diagnosis and Rehabilitation Matrixes in this chapter. Go to www.forsterpt.com and www.phase-iv.net for photos of the exercises.

GENERAL RULES:

1. Attach a thick rubber band or rubber tubing to the leg of a table or sofa. Position yourself on the floor with your legs straight out in front of you.

2. Place a rolled-up towel under your fully extended knee and another under your calf muscle, so that the ankle moves freely.

3. Perform all exercises with both ankles, even if only one is injured. This will ensure symmetry in strength and function. Perform each exercise in a pain-free range of motion only.

ANKLE DORSIFLEXION

1. Line up directly in front of the table leg with the attached rubber band. Place the band around your foot at the ball of the foot, just at the base of the toes.

2. Slide back on the floor to find a distance that puts resistance on the band with your toes pointed down.

3. Starting with the toes pointed down, keep your heel down and in place as you pivot your foot

toward your body. As the foot moves vertically toward your head, it pulls the band and exerts resistance throughout the full range of motion. All movement occurs at the ankle.

4. Release to the starting pointed-foot position. Rest for 30 seconds. Repeat, doing 10 to 20 reps.

ANKLE INVERSION

1. Position your body so that the table leg and its attached rubber band are directly to the right of your RIGHT ankle. Place the rubber band around the ball of your foot, keeping your toes pointed. Get enough distance from the table leg to create tension in the band.

2. Isolate movement of the ankle joint (you may have to hold your leg still with your hands) as you pull the right foot inward toward your left ankle as far as you can without pain.

3. Let the rubber band pull the right foot back outward as far as the ankle will permit. Perform 10 to 20 reps, rest 30 seconds, and repeat.

ANKLE EVERSION

1. Maintain your body in the same position as the Ankle Inversion, but put the rubber band around your left forefoot at the base of your toes. Keep your toes somewhat pointed down.

2. Pull the ball of your left foot to the left as far as the ankle will permit, with all movement isolated to the ankle joint. Then allow the rubber band to pull back to the right as far as the ankle will permit. Repeat 10 to 20 reps, rest for 30 seconds, and repeat.

3. Now, relocate yourself on the floor so that the rubber band and table leg are located directly to the left of your left foot. Repeat the 2 sets of Ankle Inversion with the left ankle, pulling your forefoot toward your right foot.

4. In the same position, place the rubber band around your right foot and perform Ankle Eversion by pulling your right foot to the right.

ANKLE PLANTAR FLEXION

1. Sitting on the floor, prop both legs up on rolled-up-towels under your knees and calves. Then place the rubber band around the ball of your right foot and hold the other end in your hand close to your waist, creating tension in the band.

2. Simply point your toes down, with all movement occurring in the ankle joint.

3. Then, allow the rubber band to pull your foot back up as far as your ankle will allow. Perform 20 reps, rest 30 seconds, and repeat. Repeat on your left foot.

pronation is to increase your cadence or stride frequency—that is, take more steps per minute.

Shorter, faster steps not only position your leg to land more efficiently under your center of gravity (see proper running mechanics in chapter 2), but more steps per minute translates to less time your foot spends on the ground each step. This reduces the time your foot has to pronate and limits the degree of pronation.

To limit excessive pronation related to a functional leg-length discrepancy, correct the pelvic asymmetry with the stretching and strengthening program in chapters 7 and 8. In the case of a structural leg-length problem (one leg longer than the other), use a shoe lift.

In addition to using stretching and strengthening to address long-leg mechanical deviations, use the foam roller to break up muscular adhesions, mobilize scar tissue, and help correct the dysfunctional mechanics.

If an increased cadence and leg-length correction do not alleviate the pain, then a more stable shoe with motion control and/or wearing orthotic devices in your shoes may be necessary.

Start by using the information in chapter 6 to assess your flexibility and alignment and determine whether you have a leg-length discrepancy. Then follow the rehabilitation strategies outlined in the rehabilitation grid on pages 194–195 to correct deficiencies and resolve the pain.

LEVEL OF PAIN AND DYSFUNCTION	LENGTH OF ACTIVE REHAB IN EACH LEVEL	ACTIVITY ALLOWED	FOLLOW PRICE (PROTECT, REST, ICE, COMPRESSION, ELEVATE)
LEVEL 4 · Pain outside of the knee with flat walking and squatting. · Severe pain with running.	2 weeks, then move to Level 3 rehab.	· No running for 6 weeks, then begin Walk/Run Protocol (page 166). · Stationary bike or elliptical (if not painful). Do 15–30 minutes every other day with stretching.	**P:** Get new shoes if you've run 200 miles or if you have switched to a new model of shoe recently. **R:** No running for 6 weeks, then begin Walk/Run Protocol. **I:** 3x/day for 20 minutes whether it seems to help or not. **C:** With icing 3x/day. **E:** Elevate when icing if possible.
LEVEL 3 · Pain outside of knee with running and walking up or down hills or stairs, especially after running. · Pain squatting.	2 weeks, then move to Level 2 rehab.	· No running for 4 weeks, then begin Walk/Run Protocol (page 166). · 30 minutes of stationary bike or elliptical (if not painful) every other day.	**P:** Get new shoes if you've run 200 miles or switched to a new model of shoe recently. **R:** No running for 4 weeks, then begin Walk/Run Protocol. **I:** 3x/day for 20 minutes whether it seems to help or not. **C:** With icing 3x/day. **E:** Elevate when icing if possible.
LEVEL 2 Pain during flat running.	2 weeks, then move to Level 1 rehab.	· No running for 2 weeks, then begin Walk/Run Protocol (page 166). · 30 minutes of walking 3x/week. · Stationary bike or elliptical (if not painful) every other day (for 30–60 minutes).	**P:** Get new shoes if you've run 200 miles or have switched to a new model of shoe recently. **R:** No running for 3 weeks, then begin Walk/Run Protocol. **I:** 3x/day for 2 minutes whether it seems to help or not. **C:** With icing 3x/day. **E:** Elevate when icing if possible.
LEVEL 1 · Pain after flat running. · Pain during or after running hills and speed work.	2 weeks of rehab and reduced running.	Reduce mileage by half. No speed work or hills.	**P:** Get new shoes if you've run 200 miles or switched to a new model of shoe recently. **R:** Rest 2 weeks, then begin with mileage reduced by half; stop running if pain continues. No hills or speed work. **I:** 3x/day for 20 minutes whether it seems to help or not. Continue until you are back to full pre-injury running mileage. **C:** With icing 3x/day. **E:** Elevate when icing if possible.

STATIC STRETCHING	LIGHT RESISTANCE	WEIGHTED EXERCISE	WALK/RUN
· All lower body stretches in chapter 7 (page 113), 3x/day from this day forward. · Follow Foam Roller Protocol for all lower-body muscles (page 173).	Runner's Dozen Strength Exercises (page 150). Do 3x/week. Exceptions: no squats and no bend and reach exercises.	No lower-body weight training.	· No running for 6 weeks, then begin Walk/Run Protocol. · No walking for exercise.
· All lower body stretches in chapter 7 (page 113), 3x/day from this day forward. · Follow Foam Roller Protocol for all lower-body muscles (page 173).	Runner's Dozen Strength Exercises (page 150). Do 3x/week. Exceptions: no squats and no bend and reach exercises.	No lower-body weight training.	· No running for 4 weeks, then begin Walk/Run Protocol. · No walking for exercise.
· All lower body stretches in chapter 7 (page 113), 3x/day from this day forward. · Follow Foam Roller Protocol for all lower-body muscles (page 173).	Runner's Dozen Strength Exercises (page 150). Do 3x/week. Exceptions: no squats and no bend and reach exercises.	Single-legged hamstring curl machine, seated or prone, 2 sets of 20 reps 3x/week using light weights.	Flat walking for 20 to 30 minutes 2x to 3x/week, then begin Walk/Run Protocol.
· All lower body stretches in chapter 7 (page 113), 3x/day from this day forward. Always stretch before and after every workout. · Follow Foam Roller Protocol for all lower-body muscles (page 173).	Runner's Dozen Strength Exercises (page 150). Do 3x/week and continue for at least 6 weeks until you are back to full pre-injury running.	Single-legged hamstring curl machine, seated or prone, 2 sets of 20 reps 3x/week using light weights.	· After 2 weeks of rehab, begin to build mileage by 10% to 15% per week. · No speed work or hills.

Hamstring Injuries: Anatomy and Function of the Hamstring

Strains of the hamstring, the group of three muscles on the backside of the thigh, are so prevalent among Olympic sprinters, hurdlers, and jumpers that having a reputation for being able to treat and prevent them can make a PT a rehab rock star. But the irony is that hamstring strains are not all that difficult to rehabilitate and prevent. The key is to pinpoint the precise location of the damaged tissue, reduce inflammation and scar tissue, and restrengthen the muscle.

First, an anatomy lesson: From the top, the three hamstring muscles (from medial to lateral: the semimembranosus, semitendonosis, and biceps femoris) all attach, via a common tendon, at the ischial tuberosity, the bony prominence at the base of the pelvic bone that is the contact point when we sit. At the bottom, they insert on the backside of the lower leg bone (tibia) just below the knee joint. Because the muscles of the hamstrings cross both the hip and knee joints, they are known as *two-joint muscles*.

During running, the lower part of the hamstring works in a lengthening (eccentric) contraction at the knee joint to slow down the rate at which the lower leg swings through the air before it hits the ground. At the hip, the upper part of the hamstring initially works eccentrically to limit the degree that the hip joint flexes after foot strike, which helps to slow the speed

that your center of gravity drops when your foot touches the ground. Milliseconds later, as the body moves over the foot (which is still on the ground), the hamstring muscles switch function to being active in the shortening (concentric) contraction that extends the hip joint and catapults your body weight forward over the stationary stance leg. The hamstrings, along with the glutes, are the prime movers in steady-state running on flat surfaces, because they are responsible for keeping your center of gravity moving forward. In uphill running and sprinting, they're even more active.

Hamstrings get hurt when you mistreat them in the normal way: You do too much too fast.

HOW YOU FEEL THE PAIN

Because the pain from hamstring injuries appears in different areas in the back of the leg from the glutes to behind the knee, self-diagnosis is difficult. Many runners will experience pain in the upper end of the hamstring very close to its origin at the pelvis and think they've torn the upper attachment off the bone. However, as strong as this muscle group is, it is rare that its tendon is pulled off the bone. Instead, the muscle strain is usually found about 2 to 4 inches (5 to 10 cm) below the pain itself. The difficulty in localizing the exact site of hamstring strains is further illustrated by how often a runner will come in for physical therapy evaluation complaining of a hard-to-locate pain behind the knee. After ruling out knee pathology, the pain is invariably found anywhere in a region from the midbelly of the hamstring to 4 to 6 inches (10 to 15 cm) above the knee even though the pain is experienced lower in the back of the knee.

To further complicate the hamstring pain picture, be aware that certain pain originating in the buttocks can appear in the hamstring and magnify hamstring pain. This odd effect appears when bursa, fluid-filled sacs that stop friction between the gluteus maximus and the sit bone, become inflamed and radiate pain and tightness into the neighborhood of the hamstrings. This condition, called *ischial-gluteal bursitis*, is felt as pain during sitting on both hard and soft surfaces, such as on a bench, or in stadium stands, and is typically much worse while sitting in the car. It is almost always associated with hamstring strains, but may exist in isolation, too.

If you are experiencing the pain while sitting, and it's worst when in the car, you most likely have IG bursitis. The bursitis needs to be resolved or the hamstring injury will not resolve. That's because the pain from the bursa will keep the hamstring tight. Twice-a-day stretching and icing should resolve the buttock pain. If it doesn't, see a PT who is experienced with running injuries. Also note that with hamstring strains, we do not stretch the hamstring because the scar tissue tightens on itself, like one of those Chinese finger handcuffs that tighten around your fingers when you pull the two ends apart from one another.

DIFFERENTIAL DIAGNOSIS

At least two other painful ailments can mimic a hamstring muscle strain—a compressed nerve root in the lower back (lumbar spine) and a spasm of the piriformis muscle deep in the buttock.

The piriformis is one of six "deep rotators" of the hip joint that act mostly as stabilizers during running. When a leg-length discrepancy causes a functional asymmetry, the deep rotators will often let you know it with a painful spasm that will mimic a hamstring strain. Each of these diagnoses must be ruled out by an experienced physical therapist before an isolated hamstring injury is identified and resolved.

HOW THE HAMSTRINGS GET INJURED

As the motor that powers running, hamstrings are subject to both traumatic and overuse injuries. They are highly susceptible to fatigue and a subsequent breakdown of normal function, especially because they function differently at two attachment points: the hip and the knee joint.

Overuse hamstring injuries occur from fatigue accumulated during too-long or too-hard workouts. Fatigue interferes with the hamstrings' smooth transition from a lengthening contraction to a shortening contraction, resulting in muscle-fiber and connective tissue damage, collectively known as micro-trauma. Over time, as the scar tissue that tries to repair the damage of this micro-trauma is torn and re-scarred again and again, it turns into macro-trauma, an excessive, dysfunctional scar that prevents the muscle fibers from contracting normally. Muscle fibers need to shorten and spread apart to operate normally, but the macro-scar tissue prevents this, resulting in muscle weakness that decreases performance and causes an acute strain.

As the scarred tissue accumulates, the muscle gets tighter and weaker and a dull ache will appear during or after a workout. You will lose your ability to stretch; attempts to do so only increase the muscle tightness. It turns out that the scar tissue matrix acts just like the previously mentioned Chinese finger handcuffs. This is one of the few injuries that we don't stretch in rehab—at least not until the scar tissue is resolved.

Traumatic hamstring injury is caused from overloading the hamstring and tearing a significant number of fibers all at once. The pain can be sudden and severe. Muscle strains are graded I, II, and III to indicate their severity:

A Grade I strain is caused when a limited number of fibers are disrupted. You may feel soreness after a workout and/or stiffness when you stretch. If left untreated, a Grade I strain will progress to a Grade II, which involves a more

significant portion of the muscle fibers and even more pain, and a limp home. In some instances, the damage also involves the fascia, a connective tissue sheath that wraps around the muscle belly. The acute pain of Grade II strains will make walking and performing daily activities difficult for up to 10 days or even weeks. Also, black, blue, and sometimes yellow bruising may appear farther down the thigh from the injury site 3 to 7 days postinjury as it drains through the superficial tissues.

Grade III strains involve a complete rupture of the muscle or tendon and are rare. You'll know them by an inability to contract the hamstring or walk without pain.

REHABILITATION PROGRAM

Whether you have suffered an acute traumatic muscle strain or an overuse injury, the rehab program is similar. Only the timing is different. In both instances, the inflammation must be addressed and the scar tissue has to be broken up. Finally, the muscle has to be rehabilitated to full flexibility, strength, and endurance before sport-specific workouts can begin.

In traumatic injuries the inflammation is more significant, but the focus of the first week of PRICE rehab and gentle range-of-motion exercises will begin to move the injury in the right direction. For elite athletes with an imminent competition, we will begin treating the scar tissue with cross-fiber friction massage quite early—48 to 72 hours after the injury. Cross-fiber massage is the single most important manual therapy technique used in our approach to sports injuries. This treatment involves the use of specific massage strokes applied in a direction perpendicular to the tendon or muscle fibers to disrupt the scarring that develops between fibers and prevents normal function.

To fight the lingering inflammation from the injury and limit further inflammation created with the cross-fiber massage, liberal icing and the use of ultrasound and electrical stimulation play an important role. For the recreational runner, the urgency to address the scar tissue before 72 hours is not an issue, so the PRICE acronym should guide the early phase of the rehabilitation process.

Once the acute pain and inflammation have subsided, the rehab programs for traumatic and overuse hamstring injuries proceed on the same path. In addition to cross-fiber friction massage, we instruct the injured runner to address the scar tissue with use of the foam roller and ice to control both the initial inflammation and the subsequent inflammation created by breaking up the scar tissue. To break up the scar tissue, begin by using the foam roller in the standard manner with vertical strokes from the bottom of the muscle all the way to the top, and then go back to the most tender spot; gently move your leg back and forth sideways on the roller to mimic the cross-fiber

friction massage we use in the clinic. You want to apply enough downward pressure to spread the muscle fibers apart and break up the scar tissue adhesions between the fiber.

Compression, via a wrap of self-grip tape (found in most pharmacy chain stores) or a neoprene high sleeve, not only helps resolve swelling but will support the damaged tissue and reduce pain. Light resistance exercises begin only if they can be performed without pain. Unlike rehab programs for almost all other injuries, we do not begin to stretch an injured hamstring until the scar tissue is resolved.

Once the scar tissue is cleared up, the rehabilitation program is directed at regaining full strength, flexibility, and endurance. Cross-training that can be performed without pain is introduced as tolerated to maintain fitness as the muscle is restrengthened with a progressive resistive exercise program. Only after full strength and flexibility are regained can sport-specific workouts resume.

At first, workouts consist of walking alone. They then progress to alternating between a walk and a run as you ease back into training (see pages 200–201). Mileage is increased by no more than 10 percent per week. Continue icing until you are back for full training and use the foam roller to continue to fight scar tissue, improve flexibility, and prevent re-injury.

LEVEL OF PAIN AND DYSFUNCTION	LENGTH OF ACTIVE REHAB IN EACH LEVEL	ACTIVITY ALLOWED	FOLLOW PRICE (PROTECT, REST, ICE, COMPRESSION, ELEVATE)
LEVEL 4 · Limping and/or pain with walking, especially after running. · Pain at rest, e.g., sitting, standing, and in bed. · Pain with running.	2 weeks, then move to Level 3 rehab.	· No running for 6 weeks, then begin Walk/Run Protocol (page 166). · 15 to 30 minutes of deep-water running or stationary cycling (if not painful), 3x/week.	**P:** Compress with self-grip tape or properly fit thigh sleeve. **R:** No running for 6 weeks, then begin Walk/Run Protocol. **I:** 3x/day for 20 minutes whether it seems to help or not. **C:** With icing. **E:** Elevate when icing if possible.
LEVEL 3 · Pain and/or tightness with walking, especially after running. · Pain with running.	2 weeks, then move to Level 2 rehab.	· No running for 4 weeks, then begin Walk/Run Protocol (page 166). · 30 minutes of deep-water running, stationary bike, or elliptical machine every other day for 10 minutes/week.	**P:** Compress with self-grip tape or properly fit thigh sleeve. **R:** No running for 4 weeks, then begin Walk/Run Protocol. **I:** 3x/day for 20 minutes whether it seems to help or not. **C:** With icing. **E:** Elevate when icing if possible.
LEVEL 2 · Pain and/or excessive tightness during or after running. · Stretching increases tightness.	2 weeks, then move to Level 1 rehab.	· No running for 2 weeks. · 30 minutes of deep-water running, stationary bike, or elliptical machine every other day for 10 minutes/week.	**P:** Compress with self-grip tape or properly fit thigh sleeve. **R:** No running for 2 weeks, then begin Walk/Run Protocol (page 166). **I:** 3x/day for 20 minutes whether it seems to help or not. **C:** With icing. **E:** Elevate when icing if possible.
LEVEL 1 Pain and/or excessive tightness with hills and speed work on long distances.	3 weeks of rehab and reduced mileage.	· Continue cross-training. · Flat, non-accelatory running only. No speed work or hills. · Cut daily mileage by half.	**P:** Compress with self-grip tape or properly fit thigh sleeve. **R:** No running for 2 weeks, then begin Walk/Run Protocol (page 166). **I:** 3x/day for 20 minutes whether it seems to help or not. **C:** With icing. **E:** Elevate when icing if possible.

STATIC STRETCHING	LIGHT RESISTANCE	WEIGHTED EXERCISE	WALK/RUN
All lower-body stretches in chapter 7 (page 113), except Standing Hamstring Stretch. Do 3x/day.	Runner's Dozen strength exercises (page 150) 3x/week. Exception: no squats or bend and reach exercises.	No lower-body weight training in the gym.	• No running for 6 weeks, then begin Walk/Run Protocol. • No walking for exercise.
• All lower-body stretches in chapter 7 (page 113). Do 2x to 3x/day. • Foam roller all lower-body muscles (page 172). Do once or twice a day.	Runner's Dozen strength exercises (page 150) 3x/week. Exception: no squats or bend and reach exercises.	No lower-body weight training in the gym.	• No running for 4 weeks, then begin Walk/Run Protocol. • No walking for exercise.
• All lower-body stretches in chapter 7 (page 113), 3x/day. • Foam roller all lower-body muscles (page 172), once or twice a day.	Runner's Dozen strength exercises (page 150) 3x/week. Exception: no squats or bend and reach exercises.	Single-legged hamstring curl machine, seated or prone, for 2 sets of 20 reps 3x/week, increase weight as tolerated.	Flat walking 20 to 30 minutes 2x to 3x/week, then begin Walk/Run Protocol.
• All lower-body stretches in chapter 7 (page 113), 3x/day. • Foam roller all lower-body muscles, once or twice a day. Also, continue Foam Roller Protocol (page 172).	Runner's Dozen strength exercises (page 150) 3x/week for at least 6 weeks after you are back to full pre-injury running mileage.	Single-legged hamstring curl machine, seated or prone, for 2 sets of 20 reps 3x/week, increase weight as tolerated.	• After 2 weeks of rehab begin to build mileage by 10% to 15% each week. • No speed work or hills.

About the Authors

Robert Forster, P.T., is the CEO and founder of Forster Physical Therapy and Phase IV Scientific Health and Performance Center in Santa Monica, California. He has practiced sports physical therapy (PT) for thirty-four years and lectured throughout the United States and Europe on sports rehabilitation and safety in exercise. He is the exclusive PT provider for the Los Angeles Marathon. He received his education at Stony Brook University in New York before beginning his career at the distinguished Kerlan-Jobe Orthopaedic Clinic in Los Angeles. He served as a private PT at five Olympic Games for Olympians Jackie Joyner-Kersee, Florence "Flo Jo" Joyner, Alyson Felix, and their teammates who have won a combined forty-two Olympic medals under his direct care. He has worked with pro athletes Pete Sampras, Kobe Bryant, Maria Sharapova, as well as mixed martial arts champions Joe Warren, Jay Dee "B.J." Penn, and Chael Sonnen. He has published several research studies, writes a regular column in *Triathlete* magazine, and co-authored *The Complete Water Workout Book.* Robert has served on the California Governor's Council on Physical Fitness and Sports and recently created the Herbalife 24 Fit Exercise Video for the global nutrition and weight loss company.

Roy M. Wallack is a longtime *Los Angeles Times* health section fitness-gear columnist/feature writer, a contributor to many national magazines, former editor of *Triathlete* and *Bicycle Guide* magazines, and author of many books on high-level lifelong fitness, including *Barefoot Running Step By Step*; *Bike for Life: How to Ride to 100*; *Run for Life*; *Fire Your Gym: High Intensity Workouts You Can Do at Home*; and *The Traveling Cyclist: 20 Worldwide Tours*. Over the years, Roy "broke the news" on several important fitness stories and trends that now are common knowledge, including the cycling/osteoporosis connection; the injury-reduction of the Pose Method, barefoot running, and other forefoot landing methods; the fountain-of-youth effect of all-out intervals and rapid-contraction weight training, the rise of Crossfit and high-intensity training; and the groundbreaking concept of a harmful "black hole" training zone. A former collegiate wrestler, Roy has survived some of the world's toughest endurance events, including the Himalayan 100-Mile Stage Race, the Badwater 135 UltraMarathon, the week-long Eco-Challenge and Primal Quest adventure races, the 750-mile Paris-Brest-Paris randonnee, and the mountain-bike stage races Trans-Alp Challenge, BC Bike Race, Trans-Rockies Challenge, Breck Epic, and Costa Rica's La Ruta de los Conquistadores. He finished second in the World Fitness Championship in 2004. A graduate of UCLA and Whittier College, he lives in Irvine, California.

Acknowledgments

Robert Forster: I would like to thank my science mentor, James Forster, D.D.S., who provided the spark for a life-long interest in science, and John Papalia, P.T., Ph.D., for the foundation he provided in scientific training principles for runners. Many thanks to Tom Lynn, P.T., who has always had my back at the Olympic Games. Daniel Altchuler, D.P.M., who helped launch my physical therapy practice in Santa Monica and, of course, the master coach, Bob Kersee, whose coaching techniques and competitive insight are at the core of what I provide to my clients every day. Much appreciation to the professional staff at Forster Physical Therapy and Phase IV Scientific Health and Performance Center for sharing a passion to help our clients and patients reach their highest genetic potential for injury-free performance. My mother, Madeline, for unwavering support and love through the years. Finally, I want to thank my coauthor, Roy Wallack, for making the information in this book accessible for every runner.

Index

A

Achilles tendon injuries. *See also* injuries.
 Achilles paratenonitis, 177
 Achilles tendonitis, 176–177
 Achilles tendonosis, 177
 causes of, 177–178
 eccentric contractions and, 178
 function of, 171, 176
 introduction to, 171, 176
 overpronation and, 178
 pain of, 176–177, 180
 PRICE protocol, 178–179, 180
 rehabilitation of, 178–179, 180–181
 Self-Diagnosis and Rehabilitation Matrix, 180–181
 strength training and, 181
 vulnerability of, 176
 Walk/Run Protocol, 180, 181
"adaptation" workouts, 43
addiction, running as, 20, 23
adductor muscles
 core stability and, 149
 foam roller protocol and, 174
 hip adduction strength training, 155
 standing adductor stretch, 130
 supine adductor stretch, 124
advanced glycation end products
 (AGEs), 95
aerobic exercise, 56–57, 60, 68–69
anaerobic threshold (AT), 70
ankle dorsiflexion exercise, 192
ankle eversion exercise, 192–193
ankle inversion exercise, 192
ankle plantar flexion exercise, 193
arm drills, 35
arm swing, 27–28, 115

B

barefoot running method, 26, 38
base training. *See also* Periodization
 training.
 dedication to, 42–43
 long-slow distance (LSD) running, 64
 metabolism and, 58, 60, 63–65
 nutrition and, 63, 65–66, 90
 overview, 53
 overtraining and, 42–43
 proteins and, 63, 65
 recovery and, 41–42, 65
 rushing, 40
 strength training and, 63
 structural integrity and, 66–67

body fat
 glycemic index (GI) and, 81
 insulin and, 78
 strength training and, 145
Bompa, Tudor, 40, 51
bone density, 62, 143, 164
Born to Run (Christopher McDougall), 5, 38
Boston Marathon, 4, 6
braking effect
 cadence and, 31
 heel strikes and, 26
 knee lift and, 29
 momentum and, 32
breakfast, 86
breathing, 116–117
butt kicks, 35

C

cadence
 benefits of, 30–31
 braking effect and, 31
 form and, 37
 overpronation and, 37, 38, 193
 shin splints and, 183
 treadmill and, 32
 Walk/Run Protocol and, 166
calf range of motion test, 112
carbohydrates. *See also* nutrition.
 bad carbohydrates, 84
 carbo-loading, 85
 carb-to-fat ratio, 80
 carb-to-protein ratio, 47, 93
 fats and, 80, 85–86
 fruit as, 85
 good carbohydrates, 83–84
 inflammation and, 86
 insulin and, 86
 lactate threshold (LT) and, 68
 long-slow distance (LSD) running
  and, 90
 nutritional balance and, 80
 power conversion and, 91–92
 processed carbohydrates, 85
 protein and, 84, 86, 92, 93
catback stretch, 126
center of gravity, 32, 36
Centinela Hospital Medical Center, 5
chin tuck stretch, 133
chin tuck test, 102
Chi Running method, 26
cholesterol
 inflammation and, 86
 protein and, 94
 wheat and, 94, 95
collagen
 breakdown-rebuild cycle, 143, 164, 169

connective tissues and, 61, 115,
  116, 176
 scar tissue and, 177
 stretching and, 61, 118
competition, 18
Complete Waterpower Workout Book, The
 (Lynda Huey), 50
compression clothing, 46
connective tissue
 adaptation, 61
 collagen and, 61, 115, 116, 176
 strength training and, 143, 145
Conservative Surgery (Henry Gassett
 Davis), 61
core stability
 adductor muscles and, 149
 hip abductors and, 149
 hip flexor muscles and, 148
 overview of, 148
 spine stabilization and, 148–149
 strength training and, 146, 147
cortisol, 41, 46
Cossack dance drill, 34
cross chest stretch, 134
cross-fiber massage, 199
cross-training
 injuries and, 14, 20
 Periodization training and, 76
 recovery and, 23, 54, 179

D

Davis, Henry Gassett, 61
Davis, William, 94, 95
Devers, Gail, 50
diaphragmatic breathing, 116–117
double knee-to-chest glute stretch
 test, 105
double-legged toe raises, 187

E

elevation protocol, 170
Endurox, 47
exercises
 abdominal isometric, 154
 all-fours opposite arm and leg with
  hamstring curls, 157
 alternate arms, 151
 alternate arms with knees at
  90 degrees, 152
 ankle dorsiflexion, 192
 ankle eversion, 192–193
 ankle inversion, 192
 ankle plantar flexion exercise, 193
 bracing maneuver, 150
 front plank, 158
 front plank with opposite arm and leg
  lift, 158